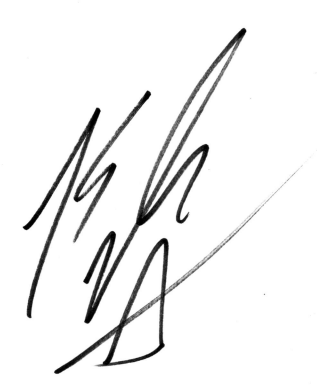

How To Maximize Your Manhood

What every red-blooded male needs to know

Clive Peters

authorHOUSE®

AuthorHouse™ UK Ltd.
500 Avebury Boulevard
Central Milton Keynes, MK9 2BE
www.authorhouse.co.uk
Phone: 08001974150

This book is a work of non-fiction. Unless otherwise noted, the author and the publisher make no explicit guarantees as to the accuracy of the information contained in this book and in some cases, names of people and places have been altered to protect their privacy.

© 2008 Clive Peters. All rights reserved.

No part of this book may be reproduced, stored in a retrieval system, or transmitted by any means without the written permission of the author.

First published by AuthorHouse 7/8/2008

ISBN: 978-1-4343-7151-5 (sc)

Library of Congress Control Number: 2008904611

This book is printed on acid-free paper.

"See, the problem is that God gives man a brain and a penis, and only enough blood to run one at a time."

..... Robin Williams

Caution

Penis enlargement, sometimes abbreviated as PE, involves techniques of tissue stretching and expanding, and other exercise routines involving the penis and/or other body parts, with and without the use of mechanical devices, and all involve some, sometimes significant, risk. You, the reader, are responsible for accepting that risk. The author, contributors, printers, publishers, distributors, and their agents, cannot be held responsible for your individual actions and will not be held liable for any damage to your health, either physical or mental, resulting from practicing penis enlargement techniques, whether as described within the pages of this book or elsewhere. The exercises described are known to increase the size of the penis if followed correctly and over time. However, as it is impossible to know of your individual state of health, we urge you to heed the cautionary notes. If you suffer from any illness, whether diagnosed before, during, or after you begin PE exercises, we cannot be held responsible. In any case, particularly if you suffer from illness of a circulatory nature, we recommend you seek advice from your qualified medical practitioner before embarking on any penile enlargement.

Sketches and technical physiological descriptions may not represent precise accuracy.

Contents

Caution vii

Foreword xiii
Trevor Roberts M.D., confirms the routines described here do work.

Preface xv
Fascination of genitalia/confidence through size/Urologists/TV and Journals.

Introduction xix
Secrets revealed/Size Does Matter/Penis Size Surveys/How to measure your penis/the first exercise.

SECTION I 1
Anatomy/The Mechanics/How do the exercises make it grow? How to begin.

SECTION II 9
Kegels/Warm-up/The Jelq/Lubrication/The OK grip/Gaining length/ Sitting/Standing/FAQs.

SECTION III 24
The First Nine Weeks/Days 5, 6, and 7/Week 2/Week 3/Fourth week/Weeks 5 and 6/Rest periods/Step back/Masturbation and making love/When to measure/Weeks 8 and 9/FAQs.

SECTION IV 36

Advanced Students/Stronger erections/Advanced stretch routines. In the bathroom/Advanced girth routines/Squeezes/Uli and Concertina. Further Research on Penis Size/ What do the Women say? Penis Enlargement Survey/ Does Penis Enlargement Work?/The Conclusion. More questions – with answers.

SECTION V 67

Hardware - Is this for me? Weights/hanging hardware and Wraps. The Theory/Penis Clamps/Method/Questions and answers on Hanging Weights.

SECTION VI 96

More Hardware Devices/Traction/Penis Extenders/Penis Pumps. Choosing the right equipment/Penis Pumps and Cylinders. Calculating dimensions/Pumping Schedule/Seven week Schedule.

SECTION VII.. 113

Using the Internet/Some Useful Websites.

SECTION VIII 117

Pills, Potions and Patches/What to believe - What not to believe. Listed Supplements.

SECTION IX... 123

...and Finally/Summary/What Urologists say.

Illustrations

Male Genitalia: external view 2

Male Reproductive Organs: cross-section 3

Penis Shaft: cross-section 4

The OK Grip 14

Power Squeezes: Uli and Concertina 52

Hanging Hardware and Wraps 71

Penis Clamps: Commercial Examples 76

Traction: Penis Extenders 97

Penis Pumps and Cylinders: Commercial Examples 103

Graphs

Penis Size Survey: Erect Penis Lengths
Respondents by Age xxvii

Average Size; before and after Penile Enlargement 62

Average Gains in Volume, related
to time spent on PE exercises 63

Foreword
By Trevor Roberts M.D.

Is there a valid medical reason to expect to get penis enlargement by the techniques listed in this book? Yes. There are cultures in the world today that teach these techniques to pubertal boys so that they attain large size as adults. 8-10 inches is the norm in length with girth of 6-8 inches.

Medically, it is simply a case of stretching skin and connective tissue and enlarging the corpus cavernosae by engorgement with blood. Stretched skin and tissue responds in two ways: there is cellular enlargement and there is replication of cells for genuine growth. This is irreversible.

If you follow the directions given in this book, you (and your partner) will notice a physical difference in length and size within a month of the time you started the programme.

Preface

Genitalia have always held a fascination for both men and women, and being dissatisfied with what you were born with is common to both sexes. There are probably as many women unhappy with the size of their breasts as there are men about the size of their penis. Two aspects of breast size are important to women: firstly, they are a physical attribute that men find attractive and their presence is difficult to ignore! Secondly, a full bosom gives a girl confidence.

For men the perceived problem is a little different; firstly, he *thinks* that the size of his penis is directly in proportion to his attractiveness to women, but the size of his manhood is always hidden by his clothing. However, if he *does* have a large penis in his pants, it gives him confidence. Put simply, find me a well endowed man and I will show you a confident one. So, for the average man, he thinks the bigger his penis can be, the better he feels about himself!

Apart from that, there's no logical reason for wanting a bigger penis and you might be disappointed to hear that in order to procreate and even give pleasure in the act, size does not matter. But, as a man, you find this difficult to accept: the man with the larger penis has always been the envy of his mates. Isn't that right? Well, maybe! But, if so, why?

Man doesn't know the answer – all he knows is that he'd be more confident not just in bed but also in everything else he does in his life. Men don't talk about these things; there's something in man's psyche that makes it difficult for him to broach the subject, just as long as he can get away with giving the impression to his peers that everything is fine in the trouser department and that the size of *his* genitals leave nothing to be desired.

Urologists will tell you that they are frequently asked if there is a way of increasing penis size. So why wish for a larger penis? What brings on the desire to do something about it? One thing is certain: we're all different! (Just how different is covered later – you will be able to compare your size with others before you start.) No matter what size you are to begin with, the research behind this book has proved to the author – and others practising the techniques described – that natural growth can be achieved without pills, potions or gadgetry. However, for those who might be interested, there is also a section describing mechanical aids that have been shown to work for many.

Returning to the *raison d'etre*, man has always felt good about himself when sexually aroused. The bigger the arousal (erection), the better he feels. The only other person to see him in this state is his lover. True, he might be seen naked in the showers at the gym but he knows that, in the flaccid state, no other man – except his partner, of course – knows what size it grows to when erect. For some though, a larger flaccid penis would send out a signal that he is just that bit 'more of a man' than the others. As I said before, he is more confident as a result.

But there are even stronger reasons for wanting a larger penis: man has always suspected that a large penis gives greater satisfaction to a woman, often refuted by women as pure nonsense. Until recent times the majority of women experienced few sexual partners, many just one in their lifetime. Nowadays it has become more common for women to have several sexual relationships before settling down to one partner; in some instances enjoying the same numbers as men are alleged to have.

Inevitably, with this wider experience, more women are discovering what it is like to have sex with a man who has a large penis – and expressing a view. There are now so many talking about it that reference to matters of size are common place. Classic examples are US TV shows like 'Sex and The City' in which story lines encourage the idea that the ideal lover is 'well hung' in the genital area.

Another show, on British TV entitled 'Am I Good In Bed?', carried out a survey with the public: they showed three women being interviewed who each stated that size was important to their enjoyment of sex. In British TV advertising, a well know French car manufacturer featured an attractive woman with a sexy French accent and snapping shut a steel measuring tape, making the simple statement that 'Size Matters.'

More recently, a day-time British TV show, 'Loose Women', featured a panel of well known female celebrities who, albeit briefly, exchanged views on the size of the male penis. One of them spoke of an engaged woman who, having discovered the size of her fiancée's penis, suggested that he 'does something about it' before they get married! Articles in women's magazines discuss the differences between men; how they look and how they perform (in bed). Even photographs featuring flaccid penises have been published – all in the name of getting the best out of relationships. (The law, at the time of writing, does not allow publication of an *erect* penis).

To illustrate there is nothing new about the views held by women, a London journal, published in the 18th Century, carried an advertisement - it actually carried a great many advertisements of this kind - by a Georgian prostitute with the following message: 'The ideal Maypole would be 9 inches. Clients are expected to pay an extra guinea for every inch they fall short of this ideal.'

There is no doubt that modern women *are* interested in the size of a man's penis, as well as all the other, and arguably more important, aspects of a relationship. Women who disclaim this as nonsense are unlikely to have experienced a larger than average penis. But, to their credit, have developed a relationship that is not built entirely on physical aspects. They also think, unless they have researched this subject, that nothing can be done about the size of a man's penis – and certainly recognise how foolish, not to say cruel, it would be to criticise a man's size. But, for the rest, there are only two ways they can find out. (Dildos are excluded from this argument because a 'relationship' with a dildo is not quite what most heterosexual women are seeking). The first is to have as many sexual partners as possible until they find a 'well endowed' man or, secondly, find their perfect partner and have him develop his penis to its optimum size and performance so that they can *both* enjoy the benefits.

Most men will be shy of sharing this new-found knowledge with a long-term partner. But, if you do share it – and you will have to at some time because she will definitely notice the changes going on – you might be surprised to learn that in all reported cases women positively encouraged their men to continue with their penile enlargement although, in most cases, they didn't want to know how the results were being achieved.

As with everything else in life, there are exceptions. The first, and surely the most obvious, is the guy who just wants a penis of gigantic proportions. For this selfish man I have only this to say: you are never going to be a thoughtful and satisfying lover. You'll only cause fright, pain and distress.

Finally, as with any physical exertion in life, you have to be fit before you set out to achieve your aims. Penile Enlargement routines are not for curing other problems. If you are suffering from any penile dysfunction, either physical or emotional, or other medical condition, you must consult with your urologist or medical practitioner before setting out on this or any other programme of physical exercises.

Introduction

Secrets Revealed

Penile enlargement, referred to from here on as 'PE', is not new. References can be found attributing an Arabic custom, originating in Persia, to the head of the family teaching his sons as soon as they reached manhood (puberty), how to 'jelq,' or 'milk', their penis to a larger size. From early teens this practice would be followed through for years, with the result that boys became men with penises of frightening proportions. Persia, during the period 550 BC to 330 BC, was one of the largest civilisations in the Western World, stretching from Libya in the West to the borders of India in the East, and there can be little doubt its cosmopolitan population was as diverse and educated as any in the world today.

It's not clear whether exercising the penis in this way was considered beneficial for sexual performance or whether to be used as an awesome sight to intimidate foes when going into battle – rather like the Scots are alleged to have done when they raised their kilts. Whatever the reason, research has not revealed any documented fact but, nonetheless, there is no doubt that PE has not only survived but, with the advent of faster and wider communications, is also gaining in numbers and popularity.

By increasing the surface area of the penis, by length and girth, there is a greater area of contact with the equally sensitive surfaces of the female's vagina. A larger penis will also have more contact with the clitoris – the female equivalent of the male penis, as a sensory member. Incidentally, the human female is the only animal on earth to be blessed with this organ; it is simply there to provide sexual stimulus and feelings of pleasure for the woman - no other purpose. Just as a man feels ready for sex when his penis becomes stretched through blood engorgement making it erect, a woman also enjoys the feeling of her clitoris being stimulated, blood engorging the tissues and making it erect, and the vagina being stretched. (Methods of getting to this point are not the subject of these pages; there are plenty of other specialist books and magazines to guide you).

There have been no clinical studies on the size of the vagina and women, like men, are not all the same. It would appear that an average size vagina is about 4 inches (10 cms) long when unexcited, or stretched. The vagina does have an enormous capability to stretch; it is, after all, the birth canal. But no man in his right mind would expect a woman to go through the equivalent of birth pains in order to take his unreasonably sized penis! I mention this because you should realise that it is not just unfair: seeing a large penis can also be intimidating for a woman – and put her completely off any of the intentions you may have had.

This is another aspect where manual PE is advantageous, especially for those already in an established relationship. There is no sudden change; growth is over time and gives both partners the opportunity to experience new feelings without the introduction of major changes all at once. You can stop your PE programme whenever you feel you have achieved optimum size to suit your relationship. Your gains will be permanent – you are not facing a regimen for life.

There are some aspects of PE that are common to working out at the gym: warming up, cooling down, and dedication to your goals. Time spent on a regular basis and an eye kept on the training manual. Keeping a note of what works for you and what doesn't. But there is one major difference: 'no pain, no gain' definitely DOES NOT APPLY. Follow the guidelines and you will not hurt. But if you are not fit to begin with, consider getting in good physical shape first. Being fit will only enhance your PE programme. Good circulation is the key to both physical fitness *and* penile enlargement. Of this there is absolutely no doubt. However, contrary to popular belief, your penis is not a muscle – and in this respect PE exercises are quite different to any your health fitness instructor will give you.

If you are overweight it is likely that you have fat around your pubic bone. Lose that fat and you might discover your penis is actually ½ inch (12.7 mm), or more, longer than you thought.

Age Concerns

There are no limits – at either end of the scale. Although I do have reservations about starting PE whilst a youthful body is still developing – despite the stories accredited to men of the Middle East. It might be wise to wait until 17 or 18 years of age, the time when the average male completes his natural penile growth – but there's no evidence either way. It is apparent that there are students of PE in their teens; if you are in that category there is nothing I can do to stop you if that's what you want to do, but I will urge you to take heed of the notes of caution you will read throughout this book. This goes for men of all ages, of course. Incidentally, and speaking of age, results of research carried out by Pfizer®, the well known pharmaceutical company, showed that the 'elderly' enjoy regular sex more than the youngsters ever believed – which won't come as any surprise to those senior folk reading this matter – and that natives of Spain and Italy do it more often than anyone else! If you are interested in sex and want to make the most of it, age will not concern you.

It is claimed that by the time a man reaches his fiftieth birthday his penis will have atrophied by as much as ½ an inch (12.7 mm): if you fall into this bracket you are promised your ½ inch back inside the first few weeks. For the dedicated and goal orientated man, permanent gains of 1 ½ to 2 inches (38 to 51 mm)or more in length and 1 to 2 inches (25 to 51 mm) in girth are attainable. Even greater gains are possible for those who wish to take it further but remember the comment about being a reasonable lover and not an intimidating chauvinist.

Give up that bad habit - smoking. Smoking damages blood vessels and results in poor circulation. Good blood flow is essential for strong erections. Smoking will decrease your chances of penile growth. It also affects the quality of your sperm – but that's another matter.

In this new age of metrication it might be correct to refer to dimensions in centimetres and millimetres but studies have shown that even the youth of today continue to use the traditional 'inch' when describing their favourite member. Thus, imperial measurements, as well as metric, are used within these pages.

Size Does Matter

There have been many references to matters of size in women's magazines but there was an article of particular interest published by Redbook Magazine, a US women's publication, in which it claimed nine out of ten women said that the *width* of a penis provides greater sexual satisfaction than length. The author of the study, Russell Eisenman, a professor of psychology at the University of Texas-Pan American (UTPA), gave the opinion that a penis that is thick at the base may stimulate the clitoris more during thrusting, because a thick penis may create more friction and can hit more of the clitoris than a thinner one.

What *is* the average size? Is mine a 'normal' length? These are questions all red-blooded males have asked themselves at some time. Whenever a man has the opportunity to compare with other males, he cannot resist a look. In the showers after the game, in the changing room, wherever you think you may get a chance peek at another man's penis, you will do so. This is in no way an indication, or reflection, of your sexual orientation, it is quite normal. Every man wants to be reassured about the size of his own penis.

Is it important? Does size really matter? And if it does, why do we (apparently) differ from each other? Scientists, commissioned by the Delta Waterfoul Foundation to look into the survival rates of different mammals, studied 122 different species, including their mating habits and physiological differences. Their findings showed that while well-endowed males didn't necessarily attract females more easily, they *were* more likely to successfully impregnate their mates at the first attempt. It was considered that this was simply because their sperm was deposited closer to the egg.

The study, which included a huge range of species – but, unfortunately, not the human – discovered massive variations in the size of penis. You might think this to be an obvious discovery, but here's where it gets interesting. True, those with the biggest penis, relatively speaking, had the best chance of inseminating a female but why should they have the largest? The harshest environments produced the best-endowed animals, apparently. Those living in environments providing less frequent opportunities of getting it together with their opposite sex had to be sure they'd succeed first time – otherwise their species could die out.

In other words, evolution was dictating the size of their genitalia. For example, the walrus is better endowed because he lives in the Polar Regions, a harsh environment. One of the authors of the study, Steven Ferguson, was reported as saying that walruses had evolved to make them more likely to be successful in a single sexual encounter. The less well-endowed elephant seals, on the other hand, live in a warmer environment where populations are denser. They encounter female seals more often, so making one pregnant first time is not such a priority for the survival of the species. Could there be some parallels for the human race as it evolved in different temperate zones of the world?

Back to us humans: a survey of 4,400 men in Poland revealed that those over 6 ft (1.83 metres) tall were, statistically, more likely to be married and have children than their shorter peers. The conclusion of that survey was that, subconsciously, women think that tall men will be physically better able to care for them and their offspring. But not every man is tall, is he? And, incidentally, do bigger men have bigger penises?

Penis Size Surveys

Most men think they are probably smaller than average. Here you can see where you stand in the averages. It might help you set your own reasonable goals for length and girth; make a note of your goals. Be realistic – and don't be in too much of a hurry.

If you go to the Internet you will discover a plethora of statistics, ranging from the original, and arguably most famous, studies of sexual behaviour carried out by Alfred C Kinsey (1894-1956) and his associates to the results of studies published by WHO (The World Health Organisation). The expression 'too much information' springs to mind when trawling through the analyses: not just erect length but also regional or ethnic differences. Not just circumference (girth) but also comparisons of those measurements taken at different points along the shaft of the penis, from the base to the glans. Not just erect but flaccid dimensions, too. American Researchers William Masters and Virginia Johnson are also well known for their long term studies conducted during the years 1954-66. They made the observation that the physical size of a man is not necessarily an indication of the size of his penis. They measured the penile lengths of over 300 men and the largest organ, measuring 14 cms (5.5 inches) in the flaccid state, belonged to a slim man who was only 5ft 7in (1.7 m) tall, and the smallest, measuring 6 cms (2.4 inches), belonged to a fairly heavily built man of 5ft 11in (1.8 m).

There are many other factors to consider when making comparisons; not least the size of the sample and the numbers making up the survey. The greater the numbers the more accurate the definition of 'average' is going to be. Then the source of the studies: are they volunteers who have been individually measured by those carrying out the survey, or are they respondents to an invitation to provide self-reported measurements. The extent of surveys carried out where men are individually measured by a third party has to be limited by definition. Imagine the logistical problems of having to measure thousands, and in many different countries throughout the world. And that's only the beginning of the problem. Consider the range of differing ages, time of day, room temperature, how recently they had sex, not to mention the affect of clinical anxiety that may affect the level of rigidity.

The best surveys then, one might argue, must be those carried out in large numbers, over the Internet, using information provided by self-measuring respondents. But what about those fooling around, the braggarts and the outright liars?

The chances are that a few, a very few, will provide misleading information and they will stand out (pardon the pun) from the rest. Sheer numbers will provide a fair indication of the averages.

Analysis of Kinsey data taken from his associates' exhaustive studies in 1948 of 3,500 college males concluded that the mean erect length of these men was 6.21 inches (157 mm), with a standard deviation of 0.77 inches (19.5 mm), whilst mean erect circumference measured was 4.85 inches (123 mm) with a 0.71 (18 mm) standard deviation.

Taken from the same analysis, mean flaccid length measured 3.89 inches (988 mm), with a 0.73 inch (185 mm) standard deviation, and flaccid circumference measured an average of 3.75 inches (952 mm) with a standard deviation of 0.65 inches (165 mm). All these measurements were taken by men who measured themselves with the length being read along the top side of the penis from the pubis to the tip and the girth from around the middle of the shaft.

The majority of surveys carried out on the world-wide-web, at the time of writing, are written up in pseudo-medical terms and analyse the measurements provided by volunteers who visit their site. Analysis in such depth makes one wonder where all this analysis is leading. There are, however, studies carried out for very serious purposes: a condom manufacturer wanting to know the sizes and shapes their products should be formed for example.

Research scientists, when referring to a world-wide survey carried out for the manufacturers of Durex® condoms, explain: 'This is a serious survey. The size of the penis is a key part of the equation as to whether or not a condom fits properly. If it does, it's more likely to be used consistently and successfully.'

These scientists compared the results of erect penis length and circumference measurements. They showed that, in agreement with previous studies, there is a distribution of penis lengths and circumferences within a given population, characterized by an average value. They added: 'The further you get away from this average value, the fewer men report having penises with these sizes. So while the "mythical" well-endowed man with a very long and very wide penis does exist, there are not many of them about.'

The survey attracted 2,936 respondents: 61% aged 16-24 years, almost a quarter aged 25-34 years, and 14% aged 35 and over.

This particular survey attracted responses mainly from the United States but also from 26 other countries, including Britain, Canada and Holland. Half of those taking part in the survey said they were circumcised – not surprising with such a high response from the US

(39%, where circumcision for non-religious reasons is still carried out routinely).

The results are shown here in graphic form:

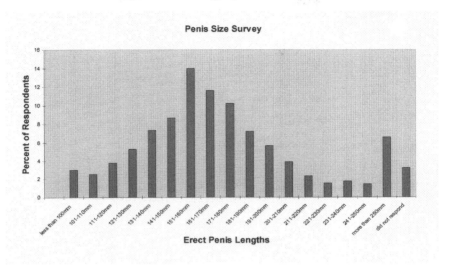

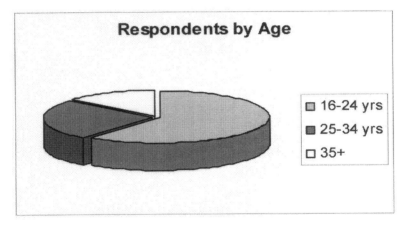

Analysing the results, the Durex team found that the average erect penis length was 6.4 inches (163 mm) with a standard deviation of 1.1 inches (28 mm). Reporting on length, around 3% of the sample measured 3.9 inches (100 mm) or less and just over 6% claimed a length of 9.8 inches (250 mm) or more. Girth, according to the analysis, is more difficult to measure, but the highest number of responses fell within the 4.76-5.1 inches (121-130 mm) grouping. The average erect circumference, at its widest point, was 5.2 inches (133 mm) with a standard deviation of 0.8 inches (21 mm). The findings also suggested that smaller than average circumferences are more common than those which are higher than the average.

As part of this survey, respondents were also asked which part of the penis was its widest point. In 42% of cases, the head of the penis was its widest point, while for 27% of men the widest point was along the shaft. A further 12% said the base of the penis was its widest point and 14% claimed their penises did not vary in width at all.

Finally, respondents were asked their views on how well condoms fit, and whether or not they had experienced problems with condom breakage or slippage. 'When it came to suggesting improvements to making condoms fit better,' say the researchers, '42% said they should be "better-shaped". There was also a clear majority in favour of increasing the width of condoms around the head of the penis. However,' they added, 'one fifth of respondents wanted nothing to change.'

All I can add is that I'm glad I don't have the responsibility of designing condoms; as I've said before, we're all different! Taking all this information into account, it is easy for us to understand the importance of such statistics in the manufacture and design of condoms. And the original reasons for penis size surveys.

How to measure your penis

Stand up; bring yourself to a full erection and, holding your penis parallel to the floor, measure from the pubis to the tip of the glans. You can locate the pubis by pressing a finger against your body at the top part of the shaft where it joins your abdomen. Using a plastic ruler will allow you to press one end against the pubis and, laying the ruler flat along the penis, enable you to read off the length.

Now measure the girth: it doesn't really matter where you take this measurement as long as, for comparative purposes, you always do it at the same point. It is generally taken at a point mid-way along the shaft whilst still erect. A tailor's cloth measuring tape is ideal but a piece of string taken around the girth and held where the end of the string meets itself then placed alongside a ruler will give you the circumference (girth) just as well.

It will be interesting to note changes in the flaccid state as well; so take these measurements the same way. On the first day make a note of these measurements in the diary you will be keeping. There are blank pages provided for such entries at the back of this book. Note-keeping is important; not just to note changes in size but also to keep a note of routines, number of repetitions (reps) and any other matters affecting your workouts, with dates, so that you can learn by looking back over your notes which exercises give best results for you.

Measuring every day is a waste of time. It's also demoralising. Measuring once a month is better – you can expect to see changes after a month's regular workouts. The speed with which you can see growth depends on you, your routine, time spent and many other variables. It also varies from one man to another – as said before, we're all different and some achieve growth faster than others. A reasonable way to look at it is that a couple of millimetres is virtually impossible to measure, but if you gained two millimetres a month, every month for a year, then you would have gained very nearly an inch in that time.

Your First Exercise

Imagine for a moment that as you read this you suddenly feel the urge to urinate but you are nowhere near a toilet. Perhaps you're in the car going to the office and you hang on for dear life because you know it'll only be a few minutes before you reach your destination and you're comforted to know there are toilets there. Why this scenario? Because you'll be doing what I'm about to describe as a fundamental necessity to the peak performance of your favourite friend. No, not squirming, but squeezing the muscle between your legs that holds everything in until you find a toilet.

This is to be your first exercise; squeeze and relax that muscle as you read this. Squeeze and maintain the squeeze for two seconds then relax. Do this ten times. Do three more repetitions of ten with just a few seconds rest in between each repetition – that's thirty in all and it will have taken you only a little over one minute. No more exercises for the moment, but read on.

From a simple exercise taking little more than a minute, within the privacy of your own pants, to a programme spread in stages over 6 months – and beyond – this book will provide answers to many questions every man, since the day he hit puberty, has pondered but rarely spoken of. The proverbial bicycle shed has seen many a fumble between the sexes and a great deal of 'old wives tales' passed on disguised as knowledge in the field of sexual matters. Women's magazines abound, writing for teens through to pensioners; relationships, pregnancy, motherhood, bringing up children, the menopause, retirement and old age. From makeovers to mud-packs, periods to panties. Agony aunts answer questions and give advice. Yes, the female sex wants to know – and is eager to learn.

There *are* men's magazines that follow the example of the ladies and you'd *expect* the subject matter to be oriented towards the male sex. It's all about how to get your girl – fair enough – and how to treat her to make sure she's satisfied, sexually that is. But, for some peculiar reason – macho springs to mind – men are happy to talk of 'conquests' but *not* of failures, especially when it relates to that set of private parts in the trousers. Well, it's time to disclose the facts, dispel the rumours, and prepare to be amazed at what you can achieve.

By the time you have read this book all the way through – and you'll probably want to keep referring back to sections as your understanding grows – you will not only appreciate what a marvellous piece of machinery you have down there but how it works, why it works, and why it sometimes doesn't. You will learn how to optimise this equipment in terms of size and performance. You will be fitter in that region than ever before. No drugs, just exercises, which you'll be happy to learn, include maintaining a healthy sex life.

It is very important that you DO NOT SKIP the first part. Indeed, if you are to become a devoted student, do not skip any part. Do not be tempted to go straight to the advanced routines without spending the recommended times on the initial exercises. There's nothing more embarrassing than turning up at A&E for emergency surgery because of self-inflicted damage to your penis. And incidentally, penis lengthening by surgery is something else your wise medical practitioner will counsel you to avoid.

The following pages will take you step-by-step through understanding your penis and the various methods of increasing its size, its performance, and you and your partner's mutual sexual pleasure. You have taken the first step; apply your new-found knowledge, feel confident and good about yourself. And your partner will love you for it.

SECTION I

Before we get on to the exercises it is important to understand how your penis functions, its construction, and how the hydraulic actions make it erect. It is a wonderful, sensitive organ, deserving care and attention. As you progress through the exercises this basic knowledge will help you to understand what is happening, to what part and why.

Anatomy

First, the bits you can see: in the unexcited, flaccid, state your penis hangs outside your body with a sack, called the scrotum, hanging beneath it. The head, or glans, of the penis has a hole through which you urinate and pass seminal fluid. 'Glans' is Latin for acorn which, if you're looking at the end of your penis with the foreskin just allowing the head to show through, does bear some resemblance. The foreskin covers the shaft and is capable of being rolled over the glans to protect it while the penis is flaccid and being free to roll back to expose the head when entering a vagina, or masturbating. For health or religious reasons

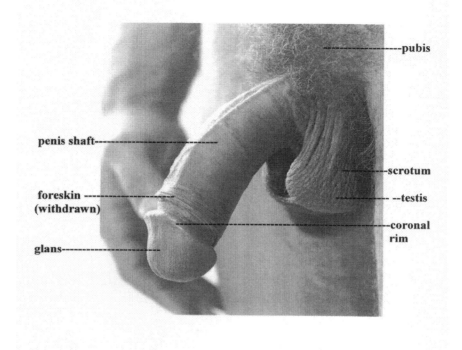

Naming the Parts

some men are circumcised and this means that sufficient foreskin has been removed so that the glans remains exposed, whether flaccid or erect. This is sometimes referred to as being 'cut' or 'uncut'. Contrary to what you might think, there is little or no difference in sensitivity between cut and uncut men.

The scrotum, the bag with the wrinkly skin, holds the testes (plural of testicle); these ARE NOT for enlarging. Do not attempt any kind of enlargement procedure with these delicate, egg-shaped, balls. However, it is possible to stretch the skin forming the scrotum so that your testes hang lower – this is covered briefly later. This is where sperm are continually produced in a myriad of tubes and, when mature, are

Male Reproductive Organs
-cross section-

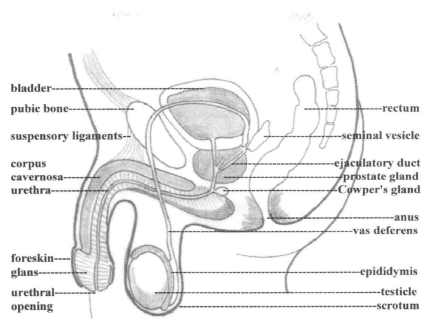

Sketches and technical physiological descriptions may not represent precise accuracy.

held in one long tube called the epididymis. Testosterone, the male hormone, is also produced by cells within the testes.

Now the bits you can't see: the urethra is the tube that ends at the tip of the penis. This connects to the bladder – the vessel that stores urine until you are ready to expel it. Situated underneath the bladder, at the point where the urethra joins it, is the prostate gland. The prostate is shaped a little bit like a doughnut and the urethra passes through the hole in the middle. This gland, along with the seminal vesicle, produces the seminal fluid that carries sperm from your body when you ejaculate. Sperm are carried through a small tube, the vas deferens, from each testicle to the prostate. It is these tubes that are severed if you undergo a vasectomy, or 'the snip' as it is commonly known. There's one more, the Cowper's gland. This gland feeds a lubricating liquid to help the flow of sperm along all these tubes as well as provide a safe saline environment for them to travel in. This is the clear liquid, rather like very fine syrup, that sometimes appears at the tip of the penis before ejaculation.

Next, the hydraulics - the parts that make a penis erect. When stimulated, by touch, sight, smell or whatever turns you on, the brain sends a signal along the nerves to open up the arteries that feed blood into your penis. Blood flows at increased pressure, up to ten times its normal rate, into the two major blood vessels that run the length of the penis shaft. The corpora cavernosa, as they are called, expand against the surrounding corpus spongiosum, making the whole shaft rigid. The penile veins that would normally allow the blood to flow back out of the penis are effectively squeezed shut by this action thus retaining the extra blood in the corpora cavernosa until another signal is sent down through the nervous system to tell the arterial blood vessels to ease up on the additional pressure. That signal is sent automatically following ejaculation.

Penis Shaft
- cross section-

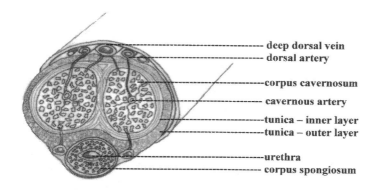

Sketches and technical physiological descriptions may not represent precise accuracy.

The mechanics

If the foregoing was all that was involved your penis would swell but remain hanging down. Penetrating a vagina would have to be assisted because there would be nothing to stop the penis from waggling around like a limb hanging on by its skin. We are now getting to the parts that not only control the rigidity of the penis and make it erect without assistance but also those same parts that will stretch allowing growth to extend length and thickness.

Surrounding these blood vessels is a tough, rubber-like mass that forms the wall of resistance to the extra blood pressure and thus making it rigid. These tissues, referred to as the tunica, extend from just behind the glans to a point close to the anus.

You will now understand that your penis is actually considerably longer than you first thought. This is what you can feel at a point halfway between your scrotum and anus – this area is described as the perineum and is, understandably, an erotic pressure point. Close to the prostate the tunica is attached to the pubic bone by ligaments. The ligaments resemble a bundle of strings reaching from the underside of the glans back to the pubic bone; at each end they fan out to provide a secure anchorage. These ligaments comprise long and short, thick and thin, lengths to make up the whole ligamentous attachment.

For the sake of comparison, imagine the penis as the boom of a crane, the vertical section from which the boom swings horizontally being your body. The ligaments are attached to the vertical section at a point above the boom and extend nearly to the end of the boom. You can imagine what would happen if you were to cut those ligaments – the surgical procedure followed by those who want their penis surgically extended. The boom – your penis – would have nothing to hold it up.

Certainly, with nothing to hold it back, all that tunica would slip forward a couple of inches, making your penis that much longer, but it would need to be lifted by hand and guided into the vagina; even then you would not have the control by body movement as you would normally because it is no longer anchored where it is needed. You will understand why I am not a fan of surgery. Ligaments can be stretched so why cut them?

How do PE exercises make it grow?

When you exercise your body you stretch tissues and ligaments, and blood circulation increases. Circulation is the key to a successful workout; blood removes carbon dioxide from the exercised tissues and expels it through the lungs. The lungs take in fresh oxygen which the blood transports back to the worked areas. Not only oxygen but also the nutrients needed for the production of new cells. This, albeit very basic, is how body builders achieve their results.

If penile enlargement is so different from body building, how can it be achieved even though it is not a muscle? As the penis doesn't have muscles to work out you have to provide that missing link – with your hands! But doesn't having an erection provide that stretch? No. Not even by masturbation? No, again. Think about it: if your penis stretched some more every time you had an erection, how long do you think it would be today?!

Body tissue stretched just a little bit more than its natural elasticity will create avulsions. An avulsion is a microscopic tear. At cellular level, it means the body will call up the necessary building blocks to create new cells at that point. As I said before, these building blocks are delivered by the blood. Continue the exercises on a regular basis and the new cells create not only flesh but blood vessels and all the other tissues essential for a working torso. So far it is no different to the body builder.

Now you can understand why, through stretching, new cells are grown and that this makes it possible to target a specific area and expect to see it grow. This doesn't mean that all you have to do is pull the life out of your penis and it will grow. No, it is not quite as simple as that, which is why you have had to plough through this pre-amble to reach the point of understanding what you are about to do. For, without a proper understanding, just as in fitness training, an uneducated move can result in damage – not something you want to do to your favourite member.

There are a number of tissues that need to be stretched at different rates: skin, blood vessels, nerves, corpora cavernosa and corpus spongiosum are all easily stretched but the tunica and ligaments don't stretch so easily.

Finally in this section, I'm going to talk about a muscle that we do have – and can exercise to advantage, everyday. The pubococcygeal muscle group (PC, for short). The PC muscle forms the 'pelvic floor' you may have heard people speak of, especially women following childbirth. It is this muscle that keeps our internal organs just that – internal. It is slung, a bit like a hammock, from front to back, with holes in it to allow the urethra, the anus and, in the case of women, the vagina to pass through. Arnold Kegel, M.D., a gynaecologist practising in the 1940s and '50s, lent his name to a simple exercise that strengthens this group of muscles. The exercise named after him, Kegel, was originally taught to women, and still is, who have had their PC muscles stretched or torn during childbirth. But it is not only women that can benefit from practising Kegels. This will be the first, and important, exercise that you will start with.

How to begin

One thing is certain: we are all different. You should recognise that PE is not a precise science. It is more like an evolving art form. 'Different strokes for different folks', certainly applies. Some men achieve gains swiftly, many take longer. Some find length easier to achieve, others girth. What you will find in the following pages are routines that are drawn from as many different men as could be found; in there is a routine for you but to start with, the basic routines are for every man.

DO NOT SKIP THE BASICS. Going straight into an advanced routine is asking for trouble – don't do it. Your penis will not be ready for it. Like training for anything, preparation is everything. Seeking medical help as a result of ignoring this advice is embarrassing at best and painful at worst.

Read and re-read the exercises. Don't be in a rush – those in a hurry do not make gains. Be dedicated. Devote a specific time and place for your regular workouts. Stick to the routines; the most frequent cause of failure to make gains is through constantly changing routines, or erratic periods of PE and rest. Keep practising – there is a learning curve but the results are rewarding if you persevere. Initial results can be expected inside the first month. From then on it is up to you – there are men out there who are devoting years to PE. The results are permanent – you do not have to be doing this for the rest of your life. It is an individual thing.

SECTION II

Kegels

Now you know what these are, here's how to do them. First you have to locate the PC muscle. When you urinate squeeze the muscle that stops the flow. That's the same as doing a Kegel. First time you visit the toilet to urinate, stop the flow a couple of times. When you can stop the flow just by flexing your PC, you are ready to practise Kegels without having to visit the urinal! Indeed, you are better off doing this exercise when you don't need to urinate; it's not fair on your bladder to interrupt the flow unnecessarily. You have identified the PC muscle and now you know how to exercise it. Do Kegels every day – any time - and do them with an empty bladder. Start gently and work up the numbers over the first couple of weeks.

Day 1 : 10 Kegels, holding each one for 2 seconds. Do this three times today.

Day 2 : 20 Kegels, holding each one for 2 seconds. Do this three times today.

Day 3 : 25 Kegels, holding each one for 2 seconds, at least three times today.

Days 4, 5 and 6 : 50 two second Kegels, twice each day.

Day 7 : 50 Kegels, holding each one for 2 seconds, three times at least.

That's the first week. If your PC muscle is in good shape you may find that you can progress to higher numbers quicker than suggested. That would be fine. You will notice that I have put a time to hold each squeeze of your PC. As you progress you will be able to hold those squeezes for longer periods. This is the way forward to gaining strength in this important muscle.

A strong PC muscle – has been referred to as the 'love muscle' – helps to make and keep erections, and a fit PC muscle gives you stronger ejaculations. Kegels aren't just for the men to practise: tell your partner about them and she'll soon realise the benefits of a fit PC muscle, too. The vagina goes through this muscle as well, so you will appreciate that the fitter her PC muscle is the firmer she can make the opening - and the grip around your penis. Something you can both benefit from straight away.

The PC muscle is quite large; sit upright on a wooden seat or any firm surface wearing only something thin and flex your PC. You will feel just how large a muscle this is between your legs. As we progress through the PE exercises there will be further mention of Kegels but the best way is to get into the habit of exercising your PC every day. Squeeze that PC every time you sit down for a meal, or every time you think of your girl friend or partner, or every time the 'phone rings; make up your own list of reminders.

Warm up – Warm down

This is an important aspect of any workout. Warming up the penis before exercising makes the tissues more pliable, stretch more readily, and gets the all-important blood flowing. You need that blood, for reasons mentioned before: to provide the hydraulic effect for expanding tissue and to bring all the nutrients straight to the places where new cells are being produced. By the way, you don't have to warm up/down for exercising the PC muscle.

What you use to warm up is up to you but here are some ideas: a hot wrap, made up of a large face-flannel or small hand towel soaked in hot water and wrapped around your penis. Wrap all the way from the tip (with foreskin drawn back if you're uncut) to allow the glans to benefit from the heat, to the abdomen so that the pubis is warmed up, too. Keep this wrap very warm by either taking it off and dipping it in the water every couple of minutes and replacing it or, provided you are standing or sitting over a bowl or basin, by pouring more hot water over the wrapped penis to maintain the temperature. Have the water at a temperature you can comfortably bear. Test it first - you don't want to scald yourself!

Another way is to simply stand at the hand basin (in the bathroom or other chosen room) filled with sufficient hot water to allow you to scoop up water with a plastic beaker (always plastic - never have glass anywhere near – broken glass is too dangerous) and continuously pour the hot water over your penis. Don't forget to have the glans exposed. Sitting on the edge of the bath, with your feet inside the bath, and holding a shower head directly onto your genitals is another way - although energy wasteful.

No hand basin? Find a plastic receptacle (tub) large enough to take the hot water and your genitals, and immerse. There are plenty of grocery items that come in a variety of tub sizes – experiment until you find one that isn't too wide to fit between your spread thighs as you sit there but deep enough to hold the water with your penis in it. The very best way is to sit in a bath of hot water filled to a point below the navel but over your genitals.

Take 5-6 minutes to get warmed up for your workout. <u>Never skip the warm up.</u> Even on rest days, when you're not working out, a five minute warm up will encourage growth through increasing circulation without stressing the tissues. When you have finished a workout it's just as important to do the same again – warm down. This not only encourages new cellular growth but also helps to avoid bruising or blood spots caused by being over enthusiastic.

The term 'cool down' is a bit of a misnomer; the cool down should be just as warm as the warm up. The best combination would seem to be a 5 minute warm up using a hot wrap and the warm down spent relaxing in a hot bath after all the exercising. The times suggested are only a guide. You might discover you need more time while you are a beginner to help keep the 'spotting' and bruising at bay and find that you can get away with less time spent warming up later in the programme. But never skip the warm up – the more intense the workout, the greater the need for the warm up. And the same goes for the warm down.

Now you are ready; you understand the terminology, you know how your penis works, you have measured up and made your first, dated, diary entry and are ready to go.

The Jelq

Jelqing describes the milking action that is the basis of all PE. You're unlikely to find the word in the dictionary but it is thought to have Arabic origins, as mentioned in the Introduction, hence the spelling without the Western European language 'u' following the 'q'. It is the basic essential exercise for all penile enlargement.

Warm up, as described earlier, then sit comfortably but upright with your knees apart and make yourself semi-erect. Don't worry if you find it difficult at first to avoid a full erection. Your penis will get used to the exercises and you will develop greater control. If it does go straight to a full erection, simply leave it alone and wait a minute. It will go down! However, if you really are having difficulty every time you touch it, go on to ejaculation, rest for 30 minutes or more and exercise after that. Learning to control is better though. An iron-hard erection is nothing like as malleable as a semi-erection. Semi-flexible might be a better description, allowing you to move the blood around inside your penis. If a full erection is described as 100% and completely flaccid as 0%, the ideal state would be around 80%. But don't dwell on this aspect too much; you will soon discover that you can quickly find the ideal state of erection.

Lubrication

You will need to lubricate your penis so that your hands can squeeze along its length without unduly dragging or pulling the skin. There are many lubricants to choose from but the simplest, most economical and readily available is baby oil. However, water based lubricants are preferable – they are easier to wash away - but some tend to dry quickly; drying gel or cream might encourage soreness but if water soluble just dip your hands in water as required to keep the lubricant slippery.

Nowadays you will find a wide choice of lubricants at your local pharmacy or superstore. Experiment and find one that you're comfortable with.

Apply a liberal amount of lube to your penis. With your dominant hand (right hand if you're right handed) make an 'OK' sign. With the

The OK Grip

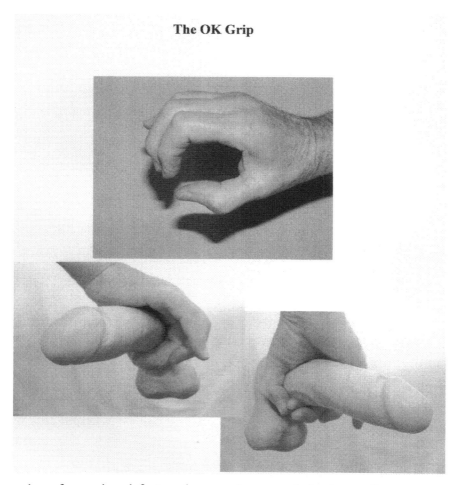

palm of your hand facing down, grip around the base of your penis with your index finger and thumb, keeping the remaining fingers gently outstretched, out of the way. You've now formed an 'OK' shape with your finger and thumb around the base of your penis and, if you've got the position right, your elbow will be pointing away from your body. Don't squeeze yet – just hold with a light grip.

Now push your hand firmly into your pubis (at the base of your penis) so that your penis is fully extended and *then* tighten your grip by closing finger and thumb together, trapping the blood in your penis. At this point you will feel your semi-erection become suddenly firmer.

Maintaining the tight grip, move your hand out along the shaft towards the glans. This action will move the trapped blood, under increasing pressure, along the shaft expanding the tissues as you go. Just before you reach the glans release the pressure and move your hand swiftly back to the base of the penis and repeat the move. If you'd like to use both hands have the other hand placed around the base ready to move up the penis as soon as you release the pressure with the first. Each of these jelqing actions should take a couple of seconds. Repeat 100 times – should take you about 3 minutes.

If you prefer to use one hand, that's fine, but change hands now and then to avoid a bias of pressure to one side only. Jelq the penis pointing slightly downwards, so that you are putting a little pressure against the upward angle that a natural erection provides.

The first day is for you to try out this basic exercise and be comfortable with it. Get comfortable with the hold so that you don't pinch or hurt yourself in any way. Use plenty of lubricant – if you are uncut (uncircumcised) you might feel more comfortable using the two-hand move described above; as the jelqing hand is moving towards the glans you use the other hand to pull the loose skin back along the shaft towards the base ready to make the next jelq. This will prevent the foreskin bunching up behind the glans – a frequent cause of foreskin bruising.

Jelqing should make you feel aware of the added pressure inside your penis and make it swell a little with each stroke – no more. If you feel a slight tingling within the penis on each jelq, that's a sure indication that you are creating maximum pressure and stretch within the penis. Any more than just a slight tingle and you are over-doing it. Remember, pain is not what we are looking for. Take it easy for the first few weeks; after a month you can start applying more intensity to your jelqing – don't worry, I'll tell you how when the time comes. Finish your jelqing sessions with a shake-out. Hold your penis at the base, between finger and thumb, and jiggle it like a snake. This will loosen up the ligaments and tunica and get the whole machinery back to normal.

This first week practise jelq sessions no more than three or four times, spread over the week. The second week you can increase to once a day for 5 days followed by two days rest.

Gaining length

Jelqing will make gains of both length and girth but to increase the probability of gains in length most students of PE include stretches in their routine. Stretching is usually included in the same workout as the jelqing session. I only talked about jelqing first because that is the one exercise that is applicable no matter what your aims are. But if your routine is to include stretching - always done flaccid and without lubrication - it makes sense to begin your PE workout with stretches and follow on with jelqing afterwards. Once again, warm up is recommended but there are some who manage stretches without. If, like me, you prefer to play safe then warm up first. Stretching can be done sitting or standing or even lying down. Let's start by lying down.

The key to successful stretching is being relaxed. It does sound not only strange but also difficult to believe that you can be relaxed while, at the same time, be strenuously pulling on your flaccid penis. Let me explain what I mean: you can try this move while lying in bed. Lie flat on your back and relax your whole body. Now grab behind the head of your completely flaccid penis with the OK hold and slowly, yes slowly, pull it up towards your chest. You will feel an involuntary muscle holding the stretch back; don't fight it, but hold very still at that point – and concentrate on relaxing again. The muscle that tightened will yield – it'll let go and allow you to pull out some more, probably about a ¼ to ½ an inch, or whatever it takes to continue the unravelling of the ligaments that are attached to the PC muscle. Continue this gentle stretch until you feel that involuntary stop no more. Your ligaments are now at their natural full length and ready for you to apply a stretch without the influence of the PC muscle holding it back. You are now ready to apply maximum pull/stretch *with the greatest effect.*

This muscle influence is not noticeable unless you are lying down. Neither is it noticeable if you start the pull/stretch in any direction other than towards your chest. But by taking advantage of this trick you can point your penis in any direction, whilst maintaining that extension, having got it at full natural length and know that all your efforts will be applied to the ligaments without trying to overcome the strength of your PC muscle as well. You may discover, as I have noted others as claiming, that pointing towards your chest can provide a most effective stretch; more about that later.

Sitting

Sit with good posture - prevents back ache and allows blood to circulate freely. So, sitting upright, knees apart and using the OK grip with palm facing away from your body, grab your penis just behind the glans. This has to be a comfortable but secure grip because all the pulling is going to be applied from this point. If there's no foreskin to get in the way, no problem. If uncut, you should experiment holding either with the foreskin covering the glans or (and you might find this is preferable) with the foreskin drawn back. Drawn right back is preferable so that your grip is directly applied under the corona (rim) of the head, and avoids pinching the foreskin. Holding awkwardly can pinch skin causing bruising - to be avoided. Spend as much time as it takes getting comfortable with the way you hold your penis for this exercise. If you feel discomfort of any kind, stop immediately. Try holding a little closer to or a little further away from the corona of the glans. When in place, the glans should be sitting with no discomfort, and little pressure, within the palm of your hand. (But you won't be able to see it of course.)

This exercise is impossible with an erection - the penis must be flaccid.

All the pressure will be applied by your finger and thumb forming the OK grip around the shaft immediately behind the glans. Grip firmly. The idea is that your pull should be on the ligaments within the penis and not just the skin surrounding it. You will know the difference; if all you're doing is pulling the skin tight away from the pubis and leaving the penis behind, you're wasting your time. The head of the penis is your stopper.

If necessary, experiment by using a wrap that allows you to grip really tightly without causing any discomfort but enables you to feel the pull on the ligaments. You can try using a face-flannel, or any other thin easy-to-wrap material, to protect the glans as well as provide a good grip around the shaft of the penis.

There will, however, be some pressure on the glans, created in two ways: blood trapped by you squeezing the shaft behind it and, secondly, by your hand using it for leverage while pulling out the penis. For this reason it's important to release your grip frequently to allow circulation to return.

Stretching is carried out at various angles so that all the ligaments get the same treatment. Pulling straight out may do the job for the central bundle but you will still be held back by the shorter, and sometimes thicker, ligaments making up the fan-shaped anchorage points around the pubis. Result: no gains. That's why we have a variety of stretches. You can actually feel the main strand of ligaments. Here's how: while standing, pull your flaccid penis straight out in front of you and with your other hand run a finger tip along the upper edge of the shaft. If you press down you'll discover that your finger is actually riding along the ligament and will slip to one side or other very easily. I'll come back to this move later.

Back to where we started; you're sitting down now, with knees apart, and your dominant hand grabbing the penis in a comfortable position just behind the glans, using a very firm OK grip.

Pull the penis downwards, between your thighs, and hold it stretched there for 30 seconds. Then relax. The glans will probably be showing signs of circulation being cut off, so run your finger and thumb along your penis a couple of times to get it back. Or just wiggle it about a bit to get the circulation going. Now hold again and pull over the top of your right thigh. Hold it there for 30 seconds. Then, holding with your left hand, do the same over your left thigh.

Standing

For the next stretch you'll have to stand up. Hold firmly as before but with the penis straight out, then make a circle with the head of your penis. Imagine the root of your penis is the pointed end of a funnel and the glans is at a point somewhere around the perimeter of the open end. Now move your stretched penis around in a circle, as if it were moving around the open end of that funnel. Move round 30 circles clockwise, maintaining a good stretch all the time – that's important. Rest and encourage blood flow again. Then circle the other way around (anti-clockwise) for another 30. Rest and jiggle it as before.

The final stretch for today (and can be done either standing or sitting): hold and pull straight out in front of you, holding the stretch for 30 seconds.

Warm down. Even if you don't warm up for stretches, warming down after stretching is highly recommended – if only to treat the head of your penis kindly.

This is an excellent time for doing Kegels, while you're warming down. Incidentally, it is good to know that one of the functions of the PC muscle is to compress the arteries that carry blood to the penis when aroused, thus trapping the blood and helping considerably to keep it erect. This compression of the arteries is an involuntary action; in other words it happens without you having to think about it. You can voluntarily (on purpose) increase this effect, making your penis harder when erect, by doing a Kegel. What you are doing is clamping the blood vessels even more than is done automatically by the autonomic nervous system. These arteries pass through openings, like holes, in the pubic bone and the muscle tissue around them constricts these vessels by pressing them against the rim of the openings. You will now understand why keeping your pubococcygeal (PC) muscle fit and strong by frequent exercise is going to help you achieve harder erections and maintain them for longer. Not only that, a strong PC will increase the energy behind the expulsion of your ejaculate – another involuntary action.

Now you have completed your warm down, gently towel dry and apply a little moisturiser. It's surprising how dry the skin can become following these exercises – even though your penis has been covered with lubricant most of the time. A simple non-fragranced moisturiser will keep the skin soft and supple, and help to prevent stretch marks and soreness.

Frequently Asked Questions (FAQs)

Q. *You have described jelqing before stretching. Does it matter what order I do them in?*

A. *You can do the exercises in the order that suits you best. You might even decide to separate the two exercises to different times of the day. But if combining the two exercises in the same session it would be more convenient to stretch first so that you don't have to wash off the lubricant after doing your jelqing. And don't forget, stretches are always done while flaccid.*

Q. *I lose count of reps easily. Can I use a time period instead?*

A. *Yes. Some prefer counting, others prefer to time. If timing, simply convert the number of reps into seconds and calculate how many minutes you have to do the exercise for. I don't recommend clock-watching (it becomes boring) but a clock that produces an audible 'tick' at one second intervals can help you count without having to keep looking at the clock.*

Q. *Little red dots (or mauve/black) appear on the head of my penis after jelqing. Am I doing it wrong?*

A. *No. This does happen sometimes when starting out. They are tiny blood blisters that will go away in 24 hours or so. Don't stint on the warm up or warm down as this will help to prevent blotches. As you progress you will find that your penis will get used to the exercises and blotches won't form.*

Bruises on the foreskin, however, are evidence that you're pinching the skin and so you should pay attention to methods of gripping and apply sufficient lubrication so that you don't pinch the skin.

Q. *When I start the milking movement from the base of my penis, hairs sometimes get caught up with the movement and .. ouch! How do I avoid this?*

A. *Shave! If you have particularly long pubic hair this does happen. The answer is to shave the shaft of the penis down to its root and trim back the surrounding hairs with scissors. This has not only practical benefit but also an aesthetic one. If you have been hiding your manhood under a bushel of pubic hair you will discover that a little trimming as described will make your penis look so much larger even before you begin. (Note: Always take great care with scissors or shaving gear when attending to the pubic area).*

Q. *I find it difficult to grip behind the glans, for stretches, without it slipping.*

A. *Dusting with a (very) little talc might help. But make sure you wash it off completely when finished. Alternatively, you may find using a damp face-flannel, or a piece of an old tee-shirt, around and behind the glans a help to your grip.*

Q. *How do I know if I'm putting enough effort into my exercises?*

A. *A good question, because you do not want to be overdoing it yet you still want to be effective. With stretches, you should feel the pull for the entire length of your penis. Don't pull so hard that it hurts! That's just not necessary or sensible. When jelqing, a grip like a firm handshake is about right and the trapped blood creating a slight tingle inside your penis as you move along the shaft is doing the job. Begin gently and work up the intensity over the weeks and you will see the results.*

Q. *Can I do stretches while erect?*

A. *No. Only stretch or pull when flaccid.*

Q. *Can I jelq while flaccid?*

A. *Yes, but you will not achieve gains in girth, although some lengthening might result.*

SECTION III

The First Nine Weeks

The techniques for the following exercises have been fully described in the previous Sections. Re-read them if unsure and, if you have opened the manual at this page hoping to skip the foregoing, don't be mistaken; start at the beginning and skip nothing.

Week 1

Days 1, 2, 3 and 4: Warm up for 5-6 minutes.
Gently towel dry, then:
Stretches –Straight down, hold for 30 seconds
To the right, hold for 30 seconds
To the left, hold for 30 seconds
Circle clockwise for 30 seconds
Circle anti-clockwise for 30 seconds.
Take this as being **1 Set** of Stretches

Jelqing - Apply lubrication to semi-erect penis.
Jelq, for 100 strokes, or no more than five minutes.
Warm down for 5-6 minutes.
25 Kegels whilst warming down. If you can do more, that's fine.

Shake out your penis.
Gently towel dry.
Apply a little moisturising cream.

All of this routine will have taken about half an hour. The first day you will be discovering the most comfortable, and effective, ways of holding your penis and carrying out the exercises. The second day you will be feeling a little more confident about your workout. You will also be tempted to do more. **Don't!**

During these first few days your penis will be subjected to exercises never previously experienced. You must give it time to get accustomed. If you hurry or skip this very important stage, you will not make gains any faster. But you could risk damaging your favourite member – something you definitely do not want to do – by imposing stresses it is definitely not ready for at this stage. You could certainly cause bruising – which means stopping your routines for a few days to allow it to recover. You have to give it time, just as in any exercising routine, to get fit and strong enough to gain from the exercises. With this dedicated programme and diligent application you will be able to go on to the advanced routines described later – but not yet. **Don't go there yet!**

Days 5, 6 and 7:

These will be rest days. Yes, time off from your workouts is as important as the workouts themselves. Notes on rest days follow later but, for now, take my word for it – rest periods are good for your penis.

Week 2

Repeat the same routine as for Week 1 but this week you can extend your workouts to 5 days, followed by **two** rest days. Don't forget to squeeze that PC: do at least 100 Kegels during the warm down this week.

Week 3

This week we are going to increase the reps. This will be a 5 day routine followed by 2 days rest, as before; from now on 5 days on and 2 days off will be the norm, until I tell you to change.

Warm up
Stretches – Three (3) Sets. That means the same stretches as you did before but repeat each sequence 3 times. That is 3 repetitions (reps) of each 30 second movement: straight down, to the left, to the right, and circular.

Jelq: 300, or 10 minutes.
Warm down. As many 2 second Kegels as you can do during warm down.
Shake out.

Week 4

The same workouts as Week 3 but **increase** the number of Jelqing strokes to 400. By now you will be falling into the routine, feeling comfortable with your grips and holds and happy either counting (using that clock I mentioned earlier in the FAQs) or timing your reps.

With the confidence you have gained from the programme so far you can begin to increase the intensity of your workouts this week

– but progress gradually. Listen to your penis; I know that sounds silly but what I mean is that your body, in this case your penis, will let you know when it has had enough – or if you're overdoing it. A good workout will leave you feeling satisfied and comfortable; your penis will feel heavier and larger but not in any kind of discomfort – if it's sore, or hurting in any way, you're either working too hard or you need to pay attention to your grip. Incidentally, you shouldn't be disappointed when, after an hour or so, your penis appears to go back to its original size – this is perfectly normal. What you have to remember is that the building of new tissue is definitely going on, but in tiny increments at each workout. After a few months you will appreciate the changes as well as see them staying with you during rest periods.

There are two ways of stepping up the programme: either increase intensity or increase time spent. You should know that increasing time spent doesn't always produce quicker results or, indeed, better results. Careful study of the programme *and* your own results is essential from here on. As I keep saying, we are all different and different men experience different growth at different rates. But you can be assured that, except for those who don't follow the routines or give up, you *will* see growth in both length and thickness.

This fourth week I'm going to suggest a little increase of both intensity and time; by slowing the pace of your jelqing. Yes, slow down! Make each stroke 3 seconds in duration. (Listen to the tick of the clock – so few people can count seconds accurately; I really do recommend you use a clock with a one-second tick.) Grip *very* firmly around the base of your penis and stroke forward with a more deliberate action. You will feel your penis expanding with the added pressure and if there's a slight tingling sensation within the tissues, that's fine. This is what causes the microscopic avulsions that result in new cellular growth. I have waited until this stage to describe it like this because if you had started on Day 1 with such intensity you would most certainly have ended up with blood blisters and spots galore. Even at Week 4 this can still happen; if it does, don't worry – the spots will disappear in a day or two and are unlikely to reappear as the tissues toughen up. Take a couple of rest days if this does happen. But it is important not to skimp on the warm-ups. Five minute warm-ups, even on rest days, will help the building process by encouraging circulation of fresh, nutrient rich, blood to build those new cells.

The preceding paragraph is *so* relevant to your entire penile enlargement programme; I'm going to ask you to read it again. Go on, do it now, because I want to be sure its relevance has sunk in. It certainly will when you put it into practise.

Weeks 5 and 6

The same basic routine as you have developed for Week 4. *But with a further increase in intensity.* Before I describe how to do this I will remind you how important it is that you should have *progressed* through the weeks to this point. If you have not, and think you can start at this level, you are mistaken. The whole point of the preceding weeks is to build up the strength of your penis as well as perfect your techniques so that you *can* progress. Like any other physical training programme, if you try to enter at a higher level than that devised for the beginner, you will definitely suffer – **there are no short cuts**, only embarrassing visits to the doctor if you ignore this advice. This is true for all physical training; whether it be for football, cricket, athletics or penile enlargement.

Stretches: So far you have used only one hand for your stretches. Starting this week you can add to the power of the stretch by using two. Grab your penis as before, with your dominant hand, and place your other hand over the first. Push out against the first hand with the second, going in the same direction of course. The first thing you will notice is that you'll probably need to grip harder with the dominant hand. The next thing you will realise is just how much more tension you can apply using both hands. From here on do all stretches as before but using *both* hands.

Because of the extra space taken up by using both hands you will find it easier, from the sitting position and leaning forward slightly, to pass both your hands *outside* your legs to grab the flaccid penis from beneath your thighs before joining hands around the penis head together. This will give you added power for a two-handed, straight down stretch. For the same reason you will find two-handed circles easier in the standing position with feet slightly apart.

Don't forget to rest between reps for 5-10 seconds and get the blood circulating freely around the glans again. A firm grip behind the glans that these stretches require does place a lot of pressure at this point and you need to look at the glans frequently to make sure all is well. When your stretch routine is complete your penis will benefit from a two or three minute dip in the hot water again before starting jelqing.

Jelqing: Squeeze very firmly around your semi-erect penis, as close to your abdomen as you can and, as you bring index finger and thumb to form that tight circle around the base, you will have noticed the instant greater rigidity of the shaft as the blood in the shaft becomes trapped. A three second stroke of the milking action towards the glans will provide that extra pressure required to further expand the tissues. However, you may feel that you could manage just a little more pressure. Here's how: as you grip around the base at each stroke, and immediately before you tighten your grip, flex your PC. That's right, do a Kegel. You will feel an instant increase of blood flow to the penis. Trap it straight away by tightening your grip, and then proceed as usual. There are other methods to increase pressure but I shall describe those when we get to the advanced routines.

When you have completed Week 6, take a week off. Rest periods are important. Do it. Sex, or masturbation, as required but in moderation – this is supposed to be a period for resting your penis.

Rest Periods

Is it really necessary to rest? Aren't I losing valuable growth-inducing exercise time? The answer is a definite 'yes' to rest and an equally definite 'no' to losing time. You can experiment with rest times. Some find they can continue their workouts 7 days a week, 30 days a month, with no breaks at all. However, I don't think this is to be recommended. A physiotherapist will tell you that tissues and ligaments need as much rest time as they do exercise. When you stop to think about it, it's quite logical. Top athletes don't go straight into their Olympic best times and distances; they build up to it, over time, and gradually – with rest periods in between. As with all your routines, plan your rest periods. They should form part of your measured overall PE programme. Don't forget to keep notes.

Resting time is when growth occurs; new cells taking up those spaces created by the stretching – in all directions. One or two days a week; weekends make good rest periods but it really doesn't matter when you take them – just as long as you do take them, and at the same regular times.

Step back: It's beneficial to take a week off from time to time – even 2 weeks, to coincide with your annual holiday, for instance, would be a good time. Following a break of 7 days or more you will need to start up again at slightly less intensity than that which you were applying before your break. This 'step back' in intensity of your workout following a rest period is good for two reasons: firstly, to avoid blood blisters (remember the little pink and red dots on the glans?) and, secondly, it's a good point to begin re-building the intensity of your workouts from a lower level during the following days. That way you'll be able to build up the intensity once more but without the need to add even more time to your workouts.

However, rest periods of 7 days or more should not be taken more frequently than following 2 or, preferably, 3 months of workouts. Many reported failures to achieve growth have, upon analysis, shown to be due to an erratic programme of workouts; settle down to your programme and stick to it. You will notice the extra 'firmness' that new cell growth will have added during the rest period. It's a rewarding feeling – and one that those who never rest do not experience, until they do eventually take a break. It's worth mentioning at this point that many reports of failing to make gains had been down to *not* including rest periods in their programme.

There is one further tip: a daily 5 minute warm-up during rest periods helps maintain good circulation. Now you have completed the first 6 weeks, rest your penis for a week; despite what I said earlier – these are still early days.

Masturbation and Making Love

Quite naturally, this is uppermost in most men's minds! But what has it to do with PE routines? When starting out on a PE programme such as this, most men want to know whether they can continue a normal sexual relationship with their partner and/or continue masturbating as frequently as they did before. It's true to say that the flow of endorphins you experience during these workouts makes you feel good – and sexy. So the temptation will always be there.

The answer probably means little or no change for most but moderation will help. Firstly, masturbation is good for your penis – as is coital sex. Both help maintain a healthy penis; keep the blood vessels supple and clear and prevent atrophy (shrinking) through lack of use. The adage 'Use it or lose it' does apply. (Another benefit of PE: these routines might help in the recovery of lost ability, as well as gains). But different men have different needs – and some need a lot more sex than two or three times a week. One correspondent declared that he would have a job keeping it down to two or three times *a day*, let alone a week!

You may find that jelqing leads to masturbating – stop and rest for a minute or so if that happens. In other words don't let masturbation interfere with your workouts. If you want to masturbate (or have sex with your partner) after you've completed your PE workout, that's fine. But giving the old guy a chance to recover first is preferable. The question of whether masturbation influences gains was asked in a survey amongst PE students – more details later – and a comparison was made amongst those masturbating more/less frequently and no differences came to light. But, an interesting correlation between masturbating and *ejaculation* did show. There is no medical reason for this but it appeared that those who ejaculated within an hour of their PE workout, either before or after, increased their penis size one third less than others who did not ejaculate in this way, over the same period of time (3 months). So, whether medically provable or not, it's arguable that you might be wiser not to ejaculate so close to your workouts.

As I said earlier, listen to your body; you will know if you are 'overdoing' it. The tissues of your penis get tired. A warning sign - apart from any obvious soreness – might come in the form of your erection waning before you've completed a routine. Overwork in your routines will also produce the same result. Recognise the signs and ease up.

When to measure

It's quite natural to measure as soon as you think you can detect growth. You will probably have measured several times since you started. Nothing wrong with that, except you risk disappointment if you measure too frequently. Once a fortnight is the shortest period I would suggest, but once a month is better. You can expect to see measurable changes after a month but, although there will be changes going on, some changes aren't easily measured.

Let me explain: new cellular growth can usually be detected by a feeling of increased 'heaviness' or 'density' of the penis – a sure sign that growth is happening – but not always measurable with a tape. At the end of each 4 week period take measurements and note them, with the date, in your record book - or make an entry in the space provided at the end of this book. Don't expect miracles after the first couple of weeks – but you should be able to measure a definite change after the first 4 weeks and this growth will encourage you to continue. Talking of growth, at cellular level we may be piling on the new cells but did you know that, on average, a human cell is about 20 microns wide – that is about two-hundredths of a millimetre. Scientists make such observations through a microscope - and we're using a tape measure; worth bearing that difference in mind. Growth will continue as long as you stay dedicated.

Weeks 8 and 9

During these two weeks follow the same routines that you completed in Week 6.

But remember, the first day back ease yourself into the intensity of your workout, then add more time on the following days.

The key to achieving gains is to avoid doing the same number of reps each day – that is unlikely to work as well. Each day, from here on especially, must see an increase in either the number of reps or an increase in intensity. In the next section on advanced routines – don't go there yet – you will learn more about applying greater pressures to increase the intensity. But, for now, add just a couple of minutes to your jelqing and the same for your stretches, each day. Sounds very little, but over the ten days to the end of Week 9 that will make your last workout 40 minutes longer than your workout on the first day of Week 8. See what I mean? If you're thinking 'this is going to become impossible; I can see myself doing PE non-stop every day,' don't worry, that isn't the case. In the next Section you will learn of techniques to reduce time spent but increase effectiveness at the same time.

You might be asking yourself: 'Why don't I just forget the first bit and go straight into the advanced routines?' That would be a big, big mistake. The whole point of the workouts described so far has been to build your penis up so that it can take the advanced routines and continue to grow from there – without having to devote every living moment to PE! By the time you have completed Week 9, and progressively applied the time added each day, your penis should be ready to take the more strenuous routines described on the following pages.

FAQs

Q. *I haven't got time to do all this during the day! What can I do?*

A. *Get up an hour earlier. Or go to bed an hour later. Or watch a little less TV in the evening. If you are truly determined to enlarge your penis you will <u>make</u> the time. You'll be amazed how easy it becomes when you fall into a routine. Especially when your partner notices the changes and you get encouraged to go do your workouts. However, for those who genuinely have no time to themselves, there is guidance later in the manual to help.*

Q. *Is there any reason why I shouldn't have a workout twice a day?*

A. *No. But not until you have completed the first couple of months. And then I suggest you simply break the two basics into two separate workouts. Say, stretches in the first session and jelq in the second.*

SECTION IV

ADVANCED STUDENTS

Not for Beginners

If you have turned to this page first, hoping to find a short cut to a speedy result, you've made a mistake. Heed the sub-title. The exercises described in the pages that follow are for advanced students only. If you have arrived at this point after following the programme for the last two or three months, congratulations, you are ready to move up a gear. If you've been working out for less than two months you're not ready for this section yet.

By now you will have realised that the essence of success is to progressively increase the number of reps to make sure the tissues are continuously stretched and don't just get used to new dimensions – and stay there. Most do arrive at a point when nothing new seems to be happening. We call this reaching a 'plateau'. If this happens to you, and you want further gains to those achieved at that point, don't worry.

There are methods to overcome a plateau – described later, because I don't expect you to have reached a plateau yet.

You will have also realised that if you continued to increase the number of reps using the routines described so far, you would end up exercising all day. Not a good idea. But we have been building up your penis so that greater pressures can now be applied by trying some different, and more intense, exercises applied in less time – that's the theory anyway.

Stronger Erections

This is simply taking the exercise of PC flexing (Kegels) a stage further. You should, by now, have got into the habit of flexing your PC not only while doing your warm-downs but also at various times during the day. A minimum of 250 a day is good to keep the PC fit. Making it stronger will give you stronger erections and stronger ejaculations.

First exercise: Sitting down, squeeze your PC and hold that squeeze for twenty seconds. Relax for 5 seconds then squeeze and hold for another twenty. Repeat until you find it difficult to either squeeze or hold. Do these exercises twice a day. Each day you will find it becomes easier and you will be able to do more reps. Then, instead of increasing the reps, increase the holding time – to 30 seconds. Repeat as before. When you can hold that squeeze for a full minute *and* do reps, you're starting to get somewhere.

Constant PC strengthening exercises might, eventually, enable you to achieve 'multiple' orgasms. You already know that as soon as you have ejaculated messages are sent by the brain to relax the tension applied by the PC muscle and open up the blood vessels to allow the blood to flow back out of your penis. Result: flaccid penis. You are also aware that if you don't ejaculate your erection stays with you until you do – unless you're over tired. With an immensely strong PC muscle, trained to hold as long as it takes for the orgasmic sensations to die away, it is possible to squeeze the PC so hard that it clamps shut the seminary vessels by squeezing them against the pubic bone through which they pass. Holding back the flow of ejaculate like this maintains the erection during and after the orgasmic sensation has died down. Keeping the PC clamped tight allows you to continue intercourse until the next wave of orgasmic sensations hit you when you can either continue as before or let your ejaculate fly.

NB: This is never to be considered a contraceptive method! Even if successfully achieved – and it is apparent that very few do ever reach these dizzy heights – sperm have a tendency to travel down the urethra whether accompanied by seminal fluid or not. If baby making is not what you're after, always wear a condom.

The foregoing requires the utmost control, not to mention months of training, but is arguably the most rewarding. Women are born with the ability to enjoy multiple orgasms – men have to work at it. Don't be upset if you cannot achieve this, remember few do, and those that do are more likely to be under twenty years old than over. ['The Multi-Orgasmic Man', by Mantak Chia and Douglas Abrams, HarperCollins(Thorsons) 2002, describes the Taoist method of achieving multiple orgasms for men of all ages]

ADVANCED STRETCH ROUTINES

There are a number of variations, all designed to do the same thing: stretch ligaments and tunica. Try them all and note your preferences. But once you have made a choice, stick with it for at least a month, preferably two. Employing two methods in the same workout produces results but more than two (stretching) doesn't appear to work so well, probably because less time is spent on any one stretch. Don't forget, all stretches must be done with the penis flaccid. If you find stretching leads to an erection then stop the stretches and start the jelqing exercises, or just wait until the erection subsides. Common sense should always prevail.

There are two schools of thought on whether to stretch before jelqing or the other way around. As I've said before: we're all different. Try both ways and find out which works best for you. Most students stretch before jelqing.

Strop the Ligament

This simple exercise certainly helps you to identify exactly where the ligaments run and helps in the early stages of stretching, but the pressures applied must be limited in their effect so you might like to try it out but then move on to another type of stretch. But if it works for you, great, stick with it. Standing, grip behind the penis head with one hand and pull your penis straight out and hold it there. With the thumb of the other hand, feel where the ligament joins the pubis at the base of the shaft. You will see that it runs along the top of the shaft, from root to glans. Now run your thumb along from the pubis out to the glans and back. This is the best way to discover how thick and pliable the strands of ligament are. Apply a little lubricant to your thumb and repeat as described but, this time, push down against the ligament as you run your thumb along the shaft. You will have to hold the penis out against this downwards pressure more strongly than when you were just feeling the ligament. Because of this you may discover it easier to swap hands.

If the ligament slips away from under the pressure, bend your thumb so that the ligament is bearing against the inside crook of the thumb-joint. Now you can ride the entire length of the ligament, from pubis to glans, bearing down with each stroke – in each direction – against the pull of the other hand holding the penis straight out. Each stroke should be made as forceful as possible so that you can feel the stretch. Start with ten strops (like an old-fashioned barber would sharpen his razor against a leather strop), rest, and then repeat ten times. As with all other exercises, gradually increase the reps over time.

Power Side Stretches

This is a variation of the stretches you have already been doing with reps to the left and right. Firstly, sit down, back straight, knees together, and form a hand into a fist and place it, with the back of the hand up, on top of your thigh – right fist to right thigh or vice-versa of course. Now do the same again but this time (here's the exercise) your fist will be holding really tightly onto the glans. With this fist pressed hard down onto your thigh, bring your other, free, hand across and place it, palm down, on top of the clenched fist – this is to make sure it doesn't move from that position. Now swing your knee outwards, keeping feet firmly in place, and feel the stretch. The further out towards your knee you place your fist, the greater the pull. You will notice some movement of the flesh on top of the thigh surrendering to the outward movement. You can negate this by using the palm of your free hand to drag this flesh across before placing the fisted glans on to the thigh. This is a powerful stretch and the glans will easily slip out of your fist if the hold isn't tight enough or if not completely dry. Here's where the action really begins: move your right knee, if that's the one you begin with, out to the right. You will feel the added power of the leg taking your hands – and your penis – to a maximum stretch. Hold for 5 seconds, followed by 5 reps.

Change hands and do the same over to the left thigh. In time you will be able to increase the time of each stretch and/or increase reps. As your penis increases in length you will be placing it further out along the thigh, of course, and appreciating even greater leverage.

This is a very powerful move – your thigh and leg muscles are much stronger than your hands and arms and so you will have to get the grip and thigh hold very firm, otherwise it will just slide off. The further out along the thigh towards the knee that you can hold your penis, the greater the pull. It's all down to angles and levers to provide maximum stretch with minimum effort. Check out the colour of the glans at frequent intervals and shake out periodically to maintain circulation.

Under the Thigh

This one can be done either standing up or sitting down. When standing, bend your knees as though about to squat. Grab behind the glans with your hand passed outside of leg and under thigh. Now try to stand up. You can't of course, because the thigh bears down on the wrist of the hand holding the penis – this provides the stretch. When lying flat, bend knee and pass hand outside and under thigh as before. Straighten the leg and feel the stretch. Hold this stretch for 5 seconds with 5 reps, then change hands and legs and repeat.

Over the Wrist

Worth describing here, even if you haven't got enough length to begin with, bear it in mind for when you can do this; a powerful stretch at an angle somewhere between upwards and outwards. Mike Salvini, of Matters of Size, is credited with devising this routine. In the sitting position and with the usual OK grip, palm facing down, grab behind the glans with your dominant hand and stretch the penis up towards your chest. Pass the other hand across and under your penis, raising the fingers of that hand so that you can place it onto the top of the wrist holding the penis. Lower both hands, still holding the penis, onto your lap. Your penis should now be bridging the wrist of your non-dominant hand. Try raising that wrist, whilst keeping a hold on the other wrist – and feel the powerful stretch.

Pendulum Swing

This is a good side-to-side stretch and is best done standing with feet comfortably spread apart. Hold behind the glans and while applying maximum downward stretch towards the floor, swing from thigh to thigh whilst maintaining the downward pull. Grip with one hand and add to the pull by holding the other hand over the first. Tilt your elbows out slightly until you can feel maximum stretch. Swing from side to side (like a pendulum) and count as you touch each thigh. Each complete swing should take about 2 seconds. First day do 50 swings. Then add 50 each day; that's 100 on the second day, 150 on the third and so on. About 300 swings, or 10 minutes, is good if maintaining this exercise.

Circles

You are already familiar with this stretch but I think it's an excellent exercise to include in your advanced routines. Two-handed and varying the diameter of the circles, sometimes making small circles to one side then the other, and doing the same pointing down as well as up – there's plenty of variation. You may feel a slight ache in the pubis when doing this, like a slight muscle ache, especially following a day of particularly strenuous stretching, and you will be able to concentrate small circles at aching points. A good place and time to do this routine is under the shower – no wasted time here. Five minutes of circles a day will assist any routine.

IN THE BATHROOM

Hand Basin Stretch

You are probably already using the bathroom for your workouts; but here are some that specifically use the bathroom facilities to help you out. It may sound strange but standing at the hand basin whilst warming up can be pretty boring and you will, naturally, be impatient to get on with your workout. Here's something useful you can do while you stand there – provided the height of the hand basin, and your own height, allows.

After a few minutes of warm-up you can start introducing some stretching. It's worth saying again at this point that warm up is not essential for stretching, which is handy because it means you can practice stretches in any private place. But my own preference, and ritual habit, is to warm up before *any* kind of workout – whether it's considered necessary or not. My reasoning for a warm up before stretching is that most of the time your glans will be under as much pressure as when jelqing – and you'd warm up for that. So, as a precaution, I advise that you warm up anyway.

What follows will relieve the tedium of warming up and can form part of your regular warm-up routine. Stand close to the basin so that you can hold your penis over the bowl. Half-fill the hand basin with water as hot as you can comfortably take and use a plastic beaker to dip into the water and pour over your penis. Less than two or three minutes into this and you can grip firmly behind the glans with an OK grip and pull straight out over the basin. Hold for ten seconds and relax. Pour some more hot water for 10 seconds or so, and then repeat. By the time you have been standing there for ten minutes your penis will be properly warmed up and ready for some serious stretches or go straight into a jelqing routine. If you find that stretching like this brings on an erection, go straight to jelqing. Don't worry about it – in time you will be able to control those feelings that cause erections and enjoy whatever time it takes to work out a thorough stretch routine.

Advanced Hand Basin Stretch

This exercise is only to be practised following a thorough warm-up, or as follow-on to the procedure just described. Once again, standing at the hand basin, grip firmly behind the glans with the OK hold and pull away from you as strongly as possible. In this position your penis will be over the basin. Adjust your feet so that, standing upright, the fist gripping the penis is on, or just over, the rim of the basin. Now lower your hand, still gripping tight, so that it rests on, or just inside the rim. Place your other hand over the top of the first and press down firmly to secure the hold on the rim – using the basin as an anchor to prevent you moving backwards.

Try it out and you'll see what I mean. You will discover that with just a well-placed finger joint or knuckle from either or both hands, you can maintain the necessary good grip on your penis as well as use the rim of the basin to 'hook' onto so that you are ready to introduce the big stretch.

Standing as described, penis fully stretched and held securely on the rim of the basin, gently push your bottom backwards – if you're tall enough you may even be able to bend your knees very slightly to add to this action. You will immediately discover this is almost impossible. But you will also discover the most incredibly strong stretch. The slightest body movement backwards, so easy to do, produces a greater pull than could ever be achieved by hands pulling out alone. The most difficult part is maintaining your grip. Dry hands and penis might help – have a hand-towel handy for the purpose – but a freshly washed penis, devoid of any lube, and wet with plain water, won't slip. A five second stretch like this, a few seconds rest then repeat, is probably the most effective straight-out stretch possible. With the hot water still in the basin, continue to pour over the penis shaft and glans between stretches.

A note of reassurance at this point: the ligaments are amazingly tough, there's no way you are going to pull the old guy out of its socket. But be as sure as you can that it is the ligaments you are stretching and not just the flesh around them. How can you tell if you are doing it right? When you stretch again the day following your initial stretches, you will feel a not-unpleasant ache deep in the pubis where the ligaments are anchored (as mentioned earlier). One note of caution: don't try this if the hand basin/plumbing isn't securely mounted!

The Bathtub Technique

Remember I said, when talking about warm-up routines, that the perfect place to warm up and warm down is in a bathtub. Well, here's an excellent stretch that you can practice while enjoying a hot soak. Fill the bathtub with sufficient water to just cover your genitals when you're sitting up. That way, when you lie down, your penis is still visible above the water level. Lie in the bath so that your feet are against the far end. Raise your head so that you can see what you're doing. Now lower your feet, so that they are still touching the far end but your heels are resting on the bottom. This should have the affect of raising your knees slightly so that your legs are no longer straight. Now spread your knees so that they are touching the sides of the bath.

Maintaining this position, grab behind the glans with your dominant hand and raise your penis at full stretch, pointing at the ceiling. Place the other hand so that it assists in the stretch. With both palms facing away from you, your elbows should be pointing out towards the sides of the bath. Whilst holding that stretch, lower the angle of your penis so that it is pointing towards your feet; this is the most effective direction to maximise the stretch away from the pubis. Probably the best angle you will be able to achieve comfortably will have your penis parallel to your thighs.

You should now be enjoying a strong stretch at this point but here comes the power to make it that much stronger: straighten your legs. You won't be able to actually straighten them at all, you will just notice your knees lower slightly and you will feel your bottom trying to travel back up the bath, but the extra stretch achieved this way will be tremendous. It will put all your practice holds to the test, just holding on! Maintain that position for a count of ten, and relax. Repeat until you tire – but certainly stop before your glans gets sore. There are two good things about this workout: firstly, you're in the right place for continuous warming, before, after, and at in-between rests and, secondly, you are using the most powerful muscles in the body to do the work for you.

ADVANCED GIRTH ROUTINES

As already stated, jelqing should result in gains of both length and girth but you may arrive at a point where you wish to gain more in girth than length. The following exercises put a definite emphasis on girth gains.

NB: None of the following workouts should be attempted before completing the basic programme, and even then, not without at least 10 minutes firm jelqing preceded by several minutes of effective warm-up.

In the early days of the Internet there was much exchange of ideas with PE – these exchanges continue today and, with few exceptions, participating communicants used pseudonyms to protect their identity

– no change nowadays, except the growth of websites, chat rooms, blogs and the intrusion of porn, has mushroomed. Unfortunately, this development has also encouraged many charlatans to appear and take advantage of the naive. Using the Internet is covered in a separate section but I mention it here because I'd like to pay tribute to all those dedicated practitioners of PE who were there to help and encourage, for no personal reward. They just wanted to share their discoveries. One such went under the name of 'Uli'. Uli was responsible for several of the most fundamental moves in creating successful girth exercises. He told us how to take advantage of the fact that the glans is not only the softest part of the erect penis but also the greatest reservoir of blood – blood that can be used to increase pressure in the chambers of the penile shaft simply by first trapping blood flow out with a closed grip around the base of the penis and then by applying a little pressure to the glans. Many of the following routines incorporate this action.

Squeezes

Squeezing a fully engorged penis provides that extra hydraulic pressure in the areas that the blood is forced into – just squeezing the shaft isn't going to do much; it's where and how you squeeze, and the movements of those squeezes that will make them effective. Here are a few that have proved to be effective; try them out and you will discover for yourself a routine that works for you.

Basic Squeeze

Warm up and slow jelq for not less than 10 minutes; it is essential that you prepare your penis in this way before doing any of these squeezes. Ignore this advice and you will be wasting your time because your penis will not be pliable enough to benefit from the squeezes if you do not prepare this way first. To put it another way, ignore the advice and not only will you put yourself at risk of bruising but also achieve nothing. Finish jelqing by stroking your penis to a full erection. Make the OK grip around the base of the penis using index finger and thumb, pushing your hand hard against the pubis so that your penis is extended as much as possible.

Flex your PC and you will feel that little extra blood pump into the shaft: at that moment trap the extra blood by squeezing your finger and thumb as hard as you can around the root of your penis. You are now holding as much blood inside your penis as it will take. Close the middle finger, followed by the third finger of the same hand to add to the clamping effect of that OK grip. This will increase the pressure and move some blood towards the penis head. Now move that 'clamp' up the shaft towards the glans. If you've got it right, your hand won't travel very far at all before you realise the pressure is so great that you can't move it along any further and you have to stop; maintain the pressure at that point and hold the position for a count of ten seconds. Repeat this exercise three times, with a rest in between each rep of only a second or two. That's enough for the first time.

Watch the glans and you will note the expansion – also look out for potential spotting, although by this stage in your programme it is most unlikely; treat your penis to a good warm down after squeezes. Always bear in mind that it is the tunica that you are working on and not the skin – use plenty of lubricant and don't bunch up the skin over the shaft or the foreskin itself. A good reminder, when you're not gripping properly is if you drag the skin and feel it pulling on the pubis. If that happens, start the move again with perhaps more lubricant and a modified grip. (And maybe some trimming and/or shaving of pubic hair that could be dragged along with your hand).

If the foreskin puffs up with fluid during a workout, understand that this does happen sometimes but is due to too much pressure in the wrong place – don't let it worry you though, a thorough warm down will take care of it. This is the lymphatic glands acting to produce fluid as a form of protection - medically described as an oedema.

Squeeze and Push

Even when your penis is fully erect you will have noticed that the glans remains relatively soft and pliable. We can take advantage of this – by using its pliability to squeeze the blood it is engorged with back into the shaft; another way to increase the pressure. Here's how:

Grip with one hand at the base, as for the basic squeeze, and place the palm of your other hand against the tip of the glans. Now move the OK grip out towards the glans and at the same time push against the glans with the other hand. The glans will give a little, forcing its blood content back into the shaft; you'll notice the increased pressure on the girth straight away.

Girth and Glans

A variation to the Squeeze and Push exercise is to shape the free hand into a fist and use the resultant shape made between finger and thumb of that hand to push the glans against. You can control the depth of glans penetration into the fist by simply making a tighter, or looser, shape between the thumb and first finger of the fist. If you keep your fist tight so that the glans doesn't penetrate at all, or just enough to maintain the position with just the very tip of the glans disappearing into your fist, the pressure created by moving the OK grip towards the glans and the resistance provided by your fist will expand the corona, or rim, of your glans as well. This exercise can be used to not only provide girth gains but also gains in glans diameter.

Enter the Fist

This is a powerful exercise for girth gains. Take up the same position as just described; with a well lubricated penis – this exercise is absolutely impossible without plenty of lubrication, particularly around the glans – grip your fully erect penis at the base, squeeze your PC and allow that little extra drop of blood pump into the shaft, grip very firmly to hold it there, and maintain your grip at the base with your hand hard up against the pubis so that as much of the penis shaft gets the benefit of this exercise as possible. Now make a fist with your free hand and push the glans into the fist, the fist should be just tight enough to make entry a slight squeeze. This movement will squeeze about half the blood content of the glans back down into the penis shaft. With the glans now held firmly inside your closed fist, close the finger and thumb that are now encircling the glans tight under the rim (corona). As the glans is now held firmly inside the fist and the finger and thumb tighten under the rim, clamping off the blood flow back into the glans, you will feel the sudden, and quite massive, increase in pressure within the penis shaft. The increase in pressure will be immediately sensed by your other hand gripping around the base of the shaft.

It may take you a few minutes to get the grip right and as comfortable as you can, but it is worth persevering; this exercise is effective. The first time you try it you may find that you can only hold the grip for a count of ten before releasing. You may find you can only manage three reps because the effort required can be really tiring – on the hands as well as on the penis. You will probably realise that you've been pulling faces in the effort to exert the strength needed to maintain the grip! It is such a powerful exercise, if you do it right, that you will notice immediately an increase in girth as you stroke up the shaft after just a couple of reps.

This increase in size disappears after a while but is a certain indication of where it is going after maintaining these exercises for a few months.

If you want to take this exercise a stage further, with both hands maintaining the pressure, clamp down the second and third fingers of the grip around the shaft base and feel the difference. Alternatively, move that OK grip along the shaft away from the pubis; it won't travel far but the additional pressure will be the most you can ever apply.

Power Squeezing

So far I have described palms-facing-down hand-holds. This is necessary to get the correct grip under the rim of the glans for squeezes and also to grip around the penis shaft as close to the root as possible. But, with your elbows pointing out, as these holds dictate, you can't be expected to apply maximum power. Sufficient, yes, but not as much you can when you grip with the palm facing the abdomen. As time progresses and you make length gains you may like to remember this: with the Girth and Glans exercise you can add more effective pressure by making the OK grip at the base with the palm facing the abdomen. The other hand making the fist should remain palm-down. This does mean, of course, that almost a hands-width of the shaft won't be getting the treatment – the distance between your grip and little finger - but with the thumbs of both hands now facing each other you are able to apply the strongest possible squeeze.

Concertina

I've called this the concertina because that describes the action – like bringing the two halves of the squeeze-box, or concertina, together. It means squeezing up from the pubis with the OK hand in the palm-to-abdomen position and, at the same time, pushing the glans against

Power Squeezes
- Uli and Concertina -

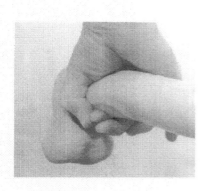

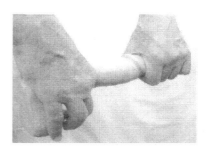

The basic Uli – above and left, with palm facing out and glans nestled against closed fist.

The Concertina, shown right, with palm facing in and glans held firmly within closed fist. Refer to text for action to increase applied pressure.

the fist of the other hand – without letting it in. This is a good squeeze for increasing glans size as well as middle shaft girth. You will feel the increase, as the pressure is immense, as soon as you've completed 2 or 3 reps of squeeze and hold each for 10 seconds.

NB: A reminder here: never go straight into an exercise like Enter the Fist, Concertina, or any power squeezing without a proper warm up period as I've described before. Always have a period of jelqing first, with plenty of lubrication handy; it will save damage and lay the foundation for growth the natural way.

PLATEAU

Reaching a plateau is the point where you don't seem to be getting any further. This is not a point where you haven't made any gains at all – that would be because you have not been following the instructions. No, this is a point that we all reach following a successful programme of workouts and suddenly realise that nothing more is happening. Workout like mad – and no further gains. Collating information on the time most reach a plateau, it seems to be 9 or 10 months into a PE programme that most students arrive at this point.

You should know that it seems quite in order to achieve gains in length ranging somewhere between 1 inch (25 mm) and 4 inches (102 mm). In some cases, even more. This isn't to say that you can set 4 inches as your goal and feel you failed because you only managed two. Be content; whatever you achieve will be the result of many months, usually a number of years in the majority of cases, of dedicated work. Be proud of your achievements and share the benefits with your partner. Don't get all hung up about 'failure'. No one who dedicates this much time and energy on self-improvement is a failure – no matter what the final result.

But that's not what you wanted to hear – right? You want more. Most correspondents during my research have been realistic about their gains. Most have partners who enjoy the size of their 'new toy'. Yes, it is not just for procreation, it is a 'plaything' between lovers. Many partners give a name, like they would a pet, to their man's penis. Both the man and his partner often refer to the penis as though it was a third party. But, yes, there are those amongst you who will never be satisfied – no matter what you gain. One correspondent replied, when asked whether he would stop PE when reaching 8 inches (203 mm): 'If 8 is great, then 9 would be fine!' He stopped at 7 ½ inches (190 mm). That's plenty for any man. He stopped because he reached a plateau at 7 ½ inches. Incidentally, that is the same man who achieved a 4 inch (102 mm) gain in length – yes, he was 3 ½ inches (89 mm) erect when he started ... nearly 4 years earlier. So the lesson is: be patient, be dedicated and if you think you have reached a plateau, think about stopping there. Your gains to that point are permanent. However, if you feel you should continue to strive for greater length and/or girth but have reached a plateau, here are some ideas for you to try.

Change of Routine

Try out a new routine; first take 7 days off working out then re-start with a completely new routine. This is where keeping notes pays off. Give it time: don't expect change inside 4 weeks – but you might measure after two weeks, just in case.

Having said that, by the time you reach this stage you will know whether gains are being made without actually measuring; you'll know by feel and experience.

Doubling Up

Try doubling up the number of periods you devote to PE. If you've been having workouts in the morning, do another workout in the evening.

Strong Stuff

If you've been cautious about applying too much pressure, give it a try for a month and see the difference. There are no gains to be had without effort.

All Three

Apply all three of the above; change the routine, double up the reps and apply greater pressure. If this routine fails to get you back into making gains, consider employing some mechanical assistance – covered later.

Take a Holiday

This may not necessarily work for you but some correspondents – myself included – have discovered that giving up PE workouts altogether for several months has enabled us to begin again and make further gains, just as though we had never practised PE before. This 'holiday' period should be 3 or 4 months at least; my own feeling is the longer the better, six months or even a year. In case you're thinking that's too long to wait, I went back to PE in order to try for greater girth, after a rest period of twelve months – and it worked. So, take heart, be patient, and know that you can always come back to it.

FURTHER RESEARCH ON PENIS SIZE

Before we consider taking our PE programme any further, it would be good to be reminded of the reasons for wanting to increase the size of our penis – to give our partners greater satisfaction? For reassurance on this point, here's some research worth reading: **Penis size: Survey of female perceptions of sexual satisfaction** Article by **Russell Eisenman**, University of Texas-Pan American, Department of Psychology, Edinburgh, TX 78539-2999 USA and published by BMC Women's Health 2001, doi:10.1186/1472-6874-1-1

Clive Peters

Background

When people speak of penis size, they typically refer to length. Thus, a man with a short but wide penis would probably think of himself as having a small penis, and would be thought so by others, too. However, width is part of size, although usually not acknowledged. Does width contribute to female sexual satisfaction? Is length more important? Or perhaps size is unrelated to female sexual enjoyment.

The famous sex researchers Masters and Johnson have concluded that size of the male penis can have no true physiological effect on female sexual satisfaction. They base this conclusion on their physiological studies that show that the vagina adapts to fit the size of the penis. Because of this vaginal adaptation, they refer to the vagina as a potential space rather than an actual space. Thus, despite the worries of many males about the size of their penis, Masters and Johnson concluded that any size penis will fit and provide adequate sexual stimulation to the female. The study reported here was conducted to see if female college students would report their sexual satisfaction related to penis length, width, or neither.

Method – Procedure

To test the notion of the possible importance of length vs. width and female sexual satisfaction, two male undergraduate college students – both popular athletes on campus – surveyed 50 female undergraduate college students, considered by the two males to be sexually active, based on the males' prior social experience and knowledge of the females.

Subjects

The female students ranged in age from 18 to 25 years old. In person or via telephone, the females were asked: 'In having sex, which feels better, length of penis or width of penis?' In half the cases, the word 'width' was used before the word 'length,' but there were no order effects. There were also no effects for telephone vs. personal interview. All female participants answered the question, perhaps because they knew the student asking the question.

Results and Discussion – what do the women say?

Of the 50 females surveyed, 45 reported that width felt better, with only 5 reporting length felt better. No females reported that they could not tell any difference. Some did report that sex in a relationship was better than sex without commitment.

Masters and Johnson have said that penis size should have no physiological effect on female sexual enjoyment, since the vagina adapts to fit the size of the penis. The current results call this conclusion into question, and point to the importance of penis width. However, Masters and Johnson could be correct if the present subjects are only reporting their psychological preference, and not showing a true physiological preference. In other words, the present study solely assessed females' perceived level of sexual satisfaction, which might differ from actual physiological arousal and satisfaction.

It is not obvious why a wide penis would be preferred to a long penis, but speculation would suggest the following. Penis width may be important due to a penis thick at the base providing greater clitoral stimulation as the male thrusts into the female during sexual intercourse. That is to say a wide penis would seem to offer a greater degree of contact with the outer part of the vagina, including the clitoral area. If this is correct, then Masters and Johnson are wrong about penis size being unrelated, physiologically, to female sexual satisfaction. Masters, Johnson, and Kolodny do not totally rule out penis size being relevant, but they suggest that it is likely of minor importance for female sexual satisfaction [see especially pages 509-510 in Masters, Johnson, and Kolodny – see ref.] Another possibility is that a wider penis provides the woman with a greater feeling of fullness, which is psychologically, and perhaps, physiologically, satisfying.

Further research on sex is necessary to understand the various influences on sexual attitudes and behaviour, including how attitudes influence behaviour if, in fact, they do. Different samples could be studied, as well as using different methods of investigation. One might have women rank different aspects of sexual satisfaction, including such things as physical attractiveness of the partner, romantic feelings, love, and other things, as well as penis size. This would give an understanding of where the different attributes rank in women's stated preferences. But width vs. length deserves study.

Conclusion

Women reported that penis width was more important for their sexual satisfaction than penis length. The results were statistically significant. Penis width needs to be given more consideration, and taken into account when one discusses penis size. Also, it may be that Masters and Johnson were wrong about penis size having little or no physiological effect on women's sexual satisfaction. However, the current data cannot provide a final answer, since they are based on self-reports of women surveyed about penis length vs. width, and their sexual satisfaction. The results reflect either a psychological preference or a true physiological reality, but we cannot say which, with the present method that was employed.

Acknowledgement and References

The author acknowledged the two reviewers, Charles Negy and Robert M Gordon. References were made to Masters WH, Johnson VE: **Human sexual response**, *Boston, Little, Brown* 1996. Masters WH, Johnson VE: **Human sexual inadequacy**, *Boston, Little, Brown* 1970. Masters WH, Johnson VE, Kolodny R: **Heterosexuality**, *New York, Harper Collins* 1994. For a full list of references please refer to the electronic version of this article which can be found on-line at: http://www.biomedcentral.com/1472-6874/1/1 © 2001 Eisenman; licensee BioMed Central Ltd.

Penis Enlargement Survey

Having considered our *raison d'etre*, the next question we'd like the answer to is: 'Are we wasting our time with penis enlargement routines?' 'Does PE work?' To find a credible answer to this question, a free-to-use on-line forum, exercisingthepenis.com, commissioned a survey of men actively practising penile enlargement routines. The author of this survey, and *Exercising The Penis*, Aaron Kemmer, first explained why results of gains were expressed as percentage gain in *volume*. It's true that we most frequently do refer to the length of a man's penis to describe *size*. And, as described in the Survey of female perceptions, it is arguable that *width* should be included in the equation when considering overall size. Thus, the aim should be, when working towards change (growth), to have an increase in girth as well as length – one dimension being in proportion to the other. Aaron Kemmer doesn't suggest what that equation might be, or should be, other than to say that a long thin penis is no more attractive than a fat, stubby penis – a balance between the two dimensions provides a pleasing aesthetic appearance; something that females, as well as males, do find attractive. And that students of PE should work on both width and length.

On this basis, enabling gains to be expressed in one figure (instead of two – length and girth), the survey was completely analysed in <u>volume</u> terms. The volume is expressed in cubic inches. For simplicity's sake, the penis was taken to be a cylindrical tube; all the little variations in shape, size of glans, and so on being ignored. If you want to calculate the volume of your penis, measure the circumference (girth) in inches and multiply that figure by itself; e.g., 5 inch girth would be 5 X 5 = 25. Now multiply that sum by the length. Let's say your penis is 6 inches long, so you multiply 25 X 6, which gives you 150. Now divide that sum by 4 X Pi (Pi = 3.1416) = 12.56. So the final sum is now 150 divided by 12.56, which equals 11.94 cubic inches. To take this example a stage further, let's assume that over a period you gained ½ inch in length and ½ inch in girth, the final equation would be 196.6 divided by 12.56 = 15.65 cubic inches. This is equal to an increase in volume of 31.1%. Remember this calculation whenever you measure progress; it will give you a greater appreciation of just what meaningful increases you are actually achieving.

The survey was advertised on the free PE forums of 'Thunders Place' and 'Matters of Size' – both on-line websites. The survey opened in April 2005, and closed in July 2005; remaining open for nearly 3 months. 957 men took The PE Survey. However, only 545 of these men completed the whole survey, and so only those men were used in the analysis. Reproduced here is a selection (only) of the summaries published from the complete survey. The author, Aaron Kemmer, stresses that the analysis should not be passed as facts; this is, after all, a survey and there is bound to be some statistical error. Further surveys are planned for the future.

The following selected points are just a few taken from the survey; a breakdown of all the results, as well as a more complete summary, can be viewed at http://www.exercisingthepenis.com/survey. [Copyright © 2005-2006 ExercisingThe Penis.com is recognised and permission to reproduce here is gratefully acknowledged].

Does Penis Enlargement work? Analysis
What did the men gain on average?
Did they believe Penis Enlargement works?

Some of the questions used in the analysis were:

Question 2: *Approximately, how long have you been using natural penis enlargement techniques, TOTAL? [For example, if you started PE'ing over 3 years ago, but only PE'd for a TOTAL of 6 months during the 3 years, then your answer would be '5-6 months.']*

Questions 6-9: *asking for PRE and POST Length and Girth: The pre and post lengths allowed* volume *to be calculated by using the formula "L X G X G divided by Pi X 4. (As explained earlier)*

Question 3: *Do you think that natural penis enlargement works? (Stretching, jelqing, and other penis exercises).*

Average Gains Analysis: Comprised of 398 men. The men that exercised their penis for less than 3 months were not included.

The Breakdown: The average gains of the 398 men were 1 inch in length, and half an inch in girth (1" X 0.51"). Translating the numbers into volume, the average pre-volume for the 398 men was 12.01 cubic inches.

The Conclusion: The 398 men increased their penis size by 42 percent. Meaning, on average, the men who exercised their penis for 3 months or more have a penis nearly half a size bigger than they started with – in terms of volume.

See Figure 1 – Average size, before and after in Cubic Inches.

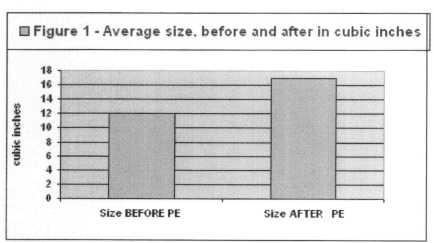

Who says Penis Enlargement doesn't work?
Question 3 asked 545 men if they think PE increases penis size. Only 7 men – approximately 1% - said 'No.'

Did the men that spent more time on a Penis Enlargement session gain more?

[It is a widely held belief that spending more time on a Penis Enlargement session increases gains. Question number 20, 'On average, how much time do you spend on a PE session?', was designed to build data on this popular assumption]

Answer choices:

10 minutes or less:	24 votes
10 to 20 mins:	99 votes
20 to 30 mins:	132 votes
30 to 45 mins:	119 votes
45 mins to 1 hour:	99 votes
1 to 2 hours:	54 votes
Multiple hours:	<u>18 votes</u>
Total voting	545 (100%)

The Breakdown: The men that spent more time on a penis enlargement session gained more. As the time spent on a penis enlargement session increased, so did the gains.

The group that spent the least amount of time on a penis enlargement session gained the least. Thereafter, the gains consistently increased with more time spent on a Penis Enlargement session.

See Figure 1. [Fig. Nos. as expressed in relevant sections of the survey.]

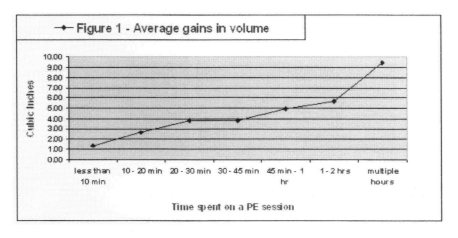

In general, most men spent 10-60 minutes on a Penis Enlargement workout. The majority of men averaged around 30 minutes per session.

The lowest gain: 10 minutes or less – gained an average of 1.36 cubic inches – an increased penis size of 10.99%. The highest gain: Multiple hours – gained an average of 9.45 cubic inches – an increased penis size of 66.46%.

Conclusion

The results from question 20 showed a correlation between increased gains and increased time spent on a PE session. According to the data, the more time spent on a Penis Enlargement session, the more gained.

The author completes this section of his survey by making these salient points: 'If you are new to penis enlargement, please take note of the following before jumping into a "multiple hours" PE session:

- Exercising the penis for multiple hours at a time, **especially in the beginning**, is a path that leads to "Injury Lane."

- Slowly increase the length of time you spend on your penis workout. In the end, anywhere from 20 minutes to an hour, 4-5 days a week, will probably give you your desired results.

The men who exercised more also had more experience, thus the increased gains were most likely a **combination** of both more time (in months/years) spent using natural penis enlargement, **and** more time spent on a Penis Enlargement session.'

The survey was summarized with brief answers to many of the questions asked. Following here are a few. On the web page from where these analyses were drawn there are links from each summary to the more detailed results of the main survey for those who might like to visit.

- **Did masturbation influence gains?** The results from Question 12 showed a strong correlation between *less masturbation* and *increased gains*. This is extremely evident when comparing the men who masturbated *once a month or less* (average gain of 6.22 cubic inches) to the men who masturbated *a few times or more* (average gain of 3.87 cubic inches). In translation, this means that the men, who masturbated once a month or less, gained 60% more cubic inches than the men who masturbated a few times a month or more.

☞ **Or was it ejaculation?** The results from Question 19 took the masturbation effect one step further, and showed no correlation between masturbation and gains among the men. However, there was a strong correlation between *less ejaculation* and *increased gains*. The group that ejaculated within an hour following a PE session increased their penis size one third less than the groups that did not. In summary, the data suggests masturbating and withholding ejaculation probably does not hurt gains, however masturbating and ejaculating *might*.

☞ **How did Penis Enlargement affect erections?** The majority of men experienced stronger and harder erection after undertaking Penis Enlargement.

☞ **Did exercising the penis cause discolouration?** Approximately 60% of the men experienced some type of discolouration after practising penis enlargement. The majority of these men reported having a darker penis; 46% overall reported having a darker penis.

☞ **Did a warm-up reduce the darkening?** There was no correlation between having a warm-up and reduced darkening.

☞ **Did a warm-up help with gains?** Using a warm-up prior to a workout had no correlation with increased gains (opposed to not having a warm-up) among the men. On average, the men that started their routine with a warm-up did not gain more than the men who did not. However, this does not mean you should throw away your heating pad (or whatever method used for warm-up). Having a warm-up is the safest known way to exercise the penis. Without a warm-up, the chances of injury are greatly increased. Additionally, a warm-up is believed to reduce the risk of bruising and other skin problems.

- **Did Penis Enlargement Pills affect gains?** The few men that used penis enlargement pills gained more than those who did not. Before you buy any 'penis enlargement pills' read the section on Pills, Potions and Patches.

- **Did exercising the penis lead to curvature?** Less than 10% of the men *noticed* a curve in their penis after practising PE.

- **Did Penis Enlargement lead to a change in erection angle?** The majority of men did not experience, or notice, any change in their erection angle after practising PE.

The most significant result of this survey, to my mind, is that it clearly demonstrates that by using only your hands you can increase the size of your penis – described as 'the natural way.' However, you might still have been thinking about getting some mechanical help to get you over a plateau, or thinking that you might make further gains with less effort and/or time. Before you do, read the next section covering these items – and take note of the cautions and disclaimers before you begin.

SECTION V

HARDWARE

Is this for me?

Your hands, and hands alone, using the techniques described so far, are all you need for penile enlargement (PE). But, human nature being what it is, and especially after a protracted period of working out using hands only, coupled with stories read and heard of dramatic gains in length and girth made by others through using weights and other mechanical aids, you will want to know the pros and cons of using weights, vacuum tubes, and various other pieces of hardware.

If I seem reticent about making recommendations in the use of mechanical aids it is partly because, in my opinion, you don't need to use them and partly because (in recognising that you might try them no matter what I say) you should understand the potential dangers of misusing them. Because I cannot see what you are getting up to in the privacy of your own home, I have to rely on you using your common sense and being totally responsible for your own actions.

It is not necessary to prove here that hanging a weight from live human tissue will make it stretch to a permanent new dimension, or putting tissue under traction will do the same. Not only do we see examples of successful traction on the necks of tribal women in Papua New Guinea, and Borneo, in the form of spiral copper rings around the neck extending them over the years by as much as 12 inches, but also native women of Central Africa putting their lips and earlobes under traction by inserting plates of ever increasing sizes to extend these parts for reasons of tribal custom. Any woman with pierced earlobes who has constantly worn heavy earrings over the years will tell you how her earlobes have extended – and remain extended when the weight of the pendant is removed.

In the West much successful surgery depends on post-surgical help with physiotherapists employing weight and traction methods to bring shortened tissue and sinews back to their required length. Remember how I described this being achieved at cellular level by avulsions? So no matter what opinions we may hold, we have to admit that hanging a weight, or putting tissue under traction, or increasing tension by placing it in a device that reduces atmospheric pressure, *does* work!

But the important aspect of this is not the fact that it works but how do you select the hardware that's right for you, and what rules do you follow to make sure you don't damage yourself? Should you go for hanging weights? Or a traction device? Or a vacuum tube? Here's a thought: it takes 3 or 4 years to train a physiotherapist, plus the time it takes for the practical experience to achieve a professional level of expertise. Bear this in mind when considering where you take your PE programme from here on.

Because the skills of practising PE are constantly evolving, and the choice of equipment in both design and range is proliferating, what follows cannot be an exhaustive appraisal but what I set out to do is demonstrate how a few pieces of equipment – that have been tried and proven to work for some – can be safely used, and the hints and tips that have been borne out of those experiences.

WEIGHTS

Light Weights

When I describe weights as 'light' they are simply to be attached and virtually forgotten about – like you might wear earrings except, in this case, it is not for visible adornment! They don't require your active involvement like other routines do. They simply hang there while you go about your daily life. There's no doubt that if you attach a weight to your penis, in time your penis will lengthen. But it's not quite as simple as that; what materials make the ideal weight? How much should it weigh? How long will I have to wear it for, and many other questions spring to mind?

Firstly, you can hang a light weight as part of your PE programme. You don't have to stop having your workouts. Indeed, hanging weights could form part of your ongoing programme, to be worn at times between workouts. All you have to do is choose a weight that can be easily and comfortably attached to your penis. Wear loose-fitting underpants that will allow the weight to hang down without being supported by any clothing - just your penis. It doesn't matter what the device is and it doesn't have to be very heavy – something around 8-10 oz (226-284 gram) will be fine to begin with.

Something small enough to be unobtrusive but with a good weight-to-size ratio – and easily attached. Brass padlocks have been widely tried; they come in a variety of sizes so you could find one to suit. To attach it to your penis you will need a broad elastic band. Put your penis through the closed padlock so that it's body hangs behind the glans, and then secure it in place with the elastic band. It should rest comfortably and not be too tight. You MUST be able to urinate without removing it – if you can't then it is definitely too tight. It will quite likely slip off the end of your penis when taking exercise, like walking. You can be assured it will only fall down your trousers at the most embarrassing moment! If you find it does slip down as you walk try adding an additional elastic band – but NEVER tighten the grip so that it restricts blood flow. That would be serious. To *guarantee* the weight won't fall down your trouser leg – even if it does slip off your penis, tie a string or cotton thread to the weight and, leaving enough slack for the weight to hang effectively, attach the other end to your belt.

An alternative device that is also available in a range of sizes/weights is the 'D' shackle, used for attaching things on boats. You can buy these in hardware stores but the best ones, in polished stainless steel – easier to keep clean and no rough surfaces to damage the skin - can be found in boat chandlers. The cheapest are made in galvanised steel and might be used for experimenting with for size and weight, but are not suitable for hanging next to the skin. So, first experiment with different sizes and then treat yourself to the more expensive, but much more comfortable and hygienic, stainless steel type of the same size.

The advantage with 'D' shackles is that you can increase weight as you feel the need, simply by adding another shackle to nestle above the first – a typical shackle would weigh about 4 oz (113 gram) so three mounted one above the next would give you 12 oz (339 gram) – and so on. Quite enough to be hanging around your trousers during a normal working day. If slippage is a real problem try using a condom. Just cut off the end and roll it on to your penis as a sleeve before mounting the weights. There are more sophisticated wraps made of clingy and stretchable materials that can be cut to size and used to protect the penis as well as provide something for the weight attachment to cling to – more on that in a moment.

Hanging Hardware & Wraps

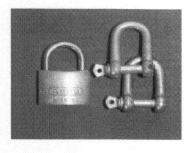

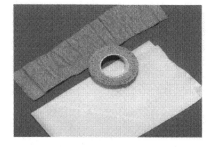

Padlocks and shackles are made In a range of sizes and weights. (See text for applications)

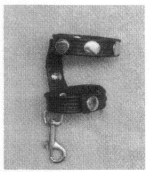

Wrapping the penis when hanging weights provides comfort and security. Examples of suitable materials are shown above.

Soft leather straps with stud Fasteners provide a secure attachment for weights. Above example by *PenisDepot.com*

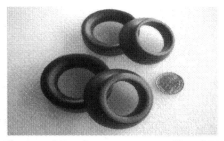

Designed for the purpose, the 'Stealth' and 'Wedge' plastic coated lead rings shown above by *PEweights.com*

Original equipment, designed for the purpose, is available through the Internet nowadays. Plastic coated lead rings, shaped for comfort, are ideal and relatively inexpensive. Illustrated are those supplied by PEweights.com; they are manufactured to different weights and sizes, and formed for comfort and ease of application. Another way of hanging light weights is to attach a strap to the penis from which a weight can be hung. Illustrated is a snap-fastener, soft leather, strap supplied by PenisDepot.com; these can be supplied either as a single, double (shown), or treble fastener strap. The advantage of multiple fasteners is that the straps can be mounted not only around the penis shaft but also completely around the penis and scrotum at the pubis; ideal for the man who wants to lower the hang of his testicles as well as lengthen his penis. The design of weight, as well as discreet attachment, is worthy of careful attention if you are to feel comfortable and confident that others are unaware that you are wearing a weight – especially when walking. Sealed sand bags are simple and can be filled to whatever weight you need. A simple ribbon or string restrainer, loosely tied around one thigh, will stop the bag from swinging around unnecessarily.

Whenever hanging a weight from the penis, the biggest problem is maintaining the grip. It should not slip down or, worse still, fall off. At the same time, it must not be fitted so tightly that it prevents you from urinating. Whatever means you choose, a simple wrap around the penis shaft before mounting the attachment is the answer; a single piece of flexible synthetic rubber sheet, or the stretchable crepe bandage that sticks to itself but not your skin, cut to size, provides the necessary comfort and grip. Both types of material are used by physiotherapists and can be purchased at pharmacies or on the web. The better weight/strap manufacturers supply such materials with their products, or as an optional extra.

The first time you dress with weights like this, check that everything is all right down there: after 15 minutes make certain that blood flow is not restricted – you'll see signs on the glans if it is – and that you can visit the toilet without any embarrassment. The first time you wear a weight remove it after 30 minutes or so and inspect your penis thoroughly. If all's well, you should be able to wear light weights like this for 6 hours or more a day, every day. Take rest days to coincide with your routine rest days. Walking is a good exercise in its own right - but walking while wearing weights provides an added advantage; the slight tug you feel with each step is what will produce the results you are looking for. But don't overdo it with the weight – the light weights I've described will be quite sufficient and shouldn't cause any problem. But don't expect instant results; employing weights like this does work but the lengthening process is very protracted. Having said that, I'm reminded that we're all different and you may discover that you're an exception; in any case, give it 3 months minimum before deciding whether to continue or not. Don't hang heavier weights than suggested in the expectation of faster results; you may get (slightly) faster results but there is a greater risk of embarrassment (it'll show) and far less comfort, not to speak of soreness.

HANGING

Heavier Weights

Great care must be observed when taking this step. DO NOT hang weights, other than described as the lighter ones, until you are at least 3, preferably 4, months into your workout programme. There is much that can go wrong – and result in devastating damage, involving loss of insensitivity through detached nerves, to causing an embolism (clot or blockage) through the wrong kind of attachment or the incorrect use of the right kind of clamp. So take note and take your time. Nonetheless, if you can devote the time – and there is no doubt that it is the *time* spent hanging weights that produces the results - you will obtain gains where other routines may have failed you.

Hanging Weights – The Theory

Whether you are interested in the mathematics or not, one way to illustrate the efficacy of your efforts in terms of weight and time spent can be expressed as lbs/minutes (or kilos/mins). Let's say you were to hang 10 lbs for 20 minutes; you multiply the weight by time spent hanging, in this example 10 X 20 = 200 lb/mins (or 90.72 kg/mins). From this equation you will quickly realize that hanging much lighter weights for considerably longer should have the same affect – maybe. Half a pound (0.23 kg) hanging for 8 hrs (480 minutes) will produce 240 lb/mins (108.86 kg/mins).

This demonstrates that less effort applied over a longer period can produce a more effective result. That could be, but what it doesn't take into account is that what works for thinner ligamentous attachments at the glans end of the shaft will have little or no effect on the thicker attachments to the pubis. That's the science. My reason for telling you this will become apparent in a minute.

Attaching a Weight

It's important that you carefully consider the method of attachment. It not only has to be strong enough to suspend the weight, it also has to be strong enough to grip your penis - safely. It is essential that it grips your penis in such a way that it doesn't tear, or bruise the tissues, nerves or blood vessels, or completely cut off the blood supply whilst, at the same time, providing maximum grip that will involve all the tissues, especially the ligaments. Not an easy task – and something that has been taxing the minds of PE practitioners for a long time. There *are* home-made designs and, for the man strapped for cash, that can be the route to go. But none are described in this book because, like fine wine, it's impossible to make your own anything like as well as can be bought from those who have spent a long time studying, researching, testing and developing their products; even taking out patents because they are so good, and manufacture devices marketed specifically for the purpose. If you read into that that I'm in favour of buying the professionally made model with a good track record, instead of a home-made version, you're right.

Penis Clamps

There are a few commercially produced products that you can find and buy on the Internet. Two are illustrated. Unfortunately, unless you have deep pockets and can afford to try them all out, you have to take your chances when deciding which would be right for you. But they are all designed to do the same job – clamp onto your penis so that a weight can hang from it. Costs are not necessarily an indication of efficiency, or ease of use, or robustness of build, not to mention practical aspects like ease of removal when in a hurry; so use your common sense: look at the pictures and make your own assessments. Also read, carefully, the notes on the website selling the product; if the design is right it will be reflected in the dialogue of the writer – he will have been a steady practitioner of PE for many years, and this will come across. Having read this book so far should help you to make a judgement. Arguably, the best will also offer free on-going practical advice and help, either direct or frequently through a forum where others can join in and share their experiences. Look around and you will recognise the examples used in these pages for illustration. They have been tried and successfully tested; both have sophisticated designs, but look hard at the designers' reasons for making them appear so different.

Attaching a Clamp

Remember what I said about the weight/time theory? Here's where hanging heavier weights takes over and where the hang-it-and-forget-it weights end, and doing what stretching by hands alone cannot do. The pull must be made closer to the thicker ligamentous attachments at the root of the penis. And the only way to do this is by clamping onto the

Penis Clamps

- Commercial examples -

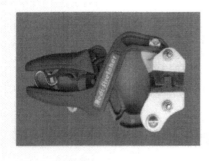 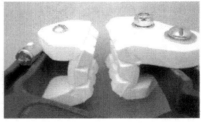

Shown at left, and with a close-up of the jaws below, is the Redi-Stretcher. *Redi-Stretcher.com*

The commercial examples shown here are both made in two sizes.

Shown below, at left and right, is The Bib Hanger. *Bibhanger.com*

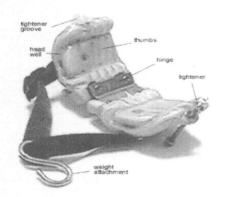 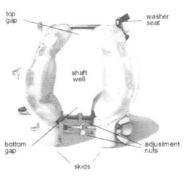

shaft, and the ligaments inside, higher up the shaft towards the pubis. This will usually mean about half-way along its length.

When you stretch using your hands, by gripping behind the glans, you are stretching the thinner ligaments and the tissues making up the shaft; that's fine, and you'll see some changes, but now we are going to stretch the thicker end at the pubis. This will not only lengthen the shaft but also add girth. Some say that stretching like this just adds length, and might even reduce thickness - not true. The new cells adding to the length are also building girth. Girth-building routines in addition to hanging will help, of course.

Essential reading - Before you begin!

It's important that you understand what you are about to embark upon. When I first thought of writing this book I contacted one of the best known characters in the PE world of hanging – known only by his correspondent name of 'Bigger'. He generously offered to share his knowledge and told me that, because hanging weights is such a individual thing, he would rather respond to questions than simply tell you what to do. Let me explain: at every stage the individual will discover aspects that he needs answers to before going any further. If all you have to refer to is a simple set of instructions you, as an individual, will find those instructions incomplete. The theory and practise is still evolving; something new is discovered all the time, whether it be relative to age, life-style, differing work-out routines, time spent, weights used and so on ... in other words, no one could possibly write a book on hanging weights that was sufficiently comprehensive to satisfy every single individual's needs. So, drawing upon his lengthy (excuse the pun) experience and effective skills, I shall set out as much as I have learnt, both from him and my own personal experience, and then finish with some of the most frequently asked questions. There are, in addition, questions that you must ask yourself. I trust that you will find the help and guidance you will need to be as safe and successful as can be.

Method – General

Don't forget the warm-up. You are about to impose greater stretching forces than your penis has ever experienced before, and warming up all the tissues, fibres, nerves and ligaments is important. Warmed up tissues not only become more flexible and stretch more readily, they also have maximum blood and lymphatic fluids flowing in them to bring those essential building blocks: new cells.

Loosen your penis by lightly stretching it by hand so that as much of the flaccid shaft is exposed as possible. NEVER ATTEMPT HANGING WHILE ERECT. Now apply a wrap to protect your penis as well as provide comfort from the pressures applied by the clamp. The best material to use is a thin synthetic rubber sheet; the kind used by physiotherapists for supporting/exercising strained ligaments. There is an excellent American product that can be bought on the Internet, described as 'Latex free' (Thera-Band®) and comes in sheets for you to cut up as required. Ask your pharmacy if they can recommend/supply a quality, thin, stretchable, synthetic rubber sheet suitable for wrapping around a limb. Now you have a sheet of this stretchable wrap, cut off a strip about 2 inches (50 mm) wide by about 15 inches (380 mm) long. The next bit is a little tricky; it would be handy if you had someone else to hold your penis out while you applied the wrap (joke) but ... with one hand stretching your penis out (this includes the foreskin if you have one), place one end of the wrap around the shaft, about 1 inch (26 mm) above the glans or even closer to the root if the length of your penis allows, and encircle the shaft just once. At this point you will just have to let go of your penis with the other hand in order to hold the wrap around the shaft. Make this first turn of the wrap as tight as possible by stretching it as you go around. You will find that, when released, the tension created by this stretching will make the rubbery surface of the wrap grip upon itself on each turn around the shaft. When you come to the end of the wrap, hold it in place ready to be captured by applying the clamp. If it makes it easier, hold the end in place with a piece of sticky tape.

It's important to make a neat job of wrapping. Don't let a fold of skin get caught while wrapping – it'll only make the whole experience uncomfortable, even painful, thus defeating the whole purpose. A good tight wrap will appear like a corset, holding the shaft in as firmly as possible, to form a smooth surface for the clamp to grip without inflicting any pain, yet still allowing blood to circulate, in and out of the penis.

There are other wrap materials you might try, like a strip cut from an old T-shirt, or even toilet tissue (not the best idea), or the crepe bandage described earlier, but the synthetic rubber sheet not only does the job well but can also be re-used over and over. Apply the wrap as high up the shaft, that is as close to the pubis, as you can without pinching the scrotal skin. Too close to the glans and you will have undue pressure put on the glans with skin piling up behind it. Practice wrapping a few times – you'll know when you've got it right. Never apply a clamp to an unwrapped penis and never apply a clamp to a shaft that does not feel completely comfortable.

You are now ready to fit the clamp. Re-read the instructions that accompany the clamp to ensure you fit it around the right way and tighten it up so that you can feel the pressure applied to the shaft. Don't attach any weight yet. Wait for 2 or 3 minutes then tighten again. Don't be in too much of a hurry with this first fitting. Remember that adjustment of the clamp not only allows you to adjust grip for tightness but also the angle between the cheeks of the grip so that you can have a degree of toe-in. Try adjusting and see what suits you best. Once adjusted you are unlikely to want to change any toe-in angle so subsequent fittings will be done in a fraction of the time. You should now feel comfortable but with maximum grip applied. Check your glans for signs of anything unusual; any signs of stress and you should immediately release the tension. Assuming all is well; attach the weight to the 'S' hook.

How much weight?

A little further on I will talk some more about the pros and cons of differing weights but, <u>to begin</u>, DO NOT hang more than a kilo (2.2 lbs). Many grocery products come in handy one kilo packets; a pack of sugar would be a good starter. Use a plastic shopping bag to place the weight in and hook its handles over the 'S' hook hanging from the clamp. If you have a set of scales, fine, you can weigh stones/rocks from the garden in a bag with the same result.

For how long should I hang?

This first time it is going to be no more than 1 kilo (2.2 lbs) – and you are going to hang for no more than 20 minutes. No argument.

First, a straight forward hang, standing upright, feet slightly apart, with the weight hanging down between your knees. Get accustomed to the feel of the stretch. Move your body slightly from side to side; feel the change in the pull on different areas of the pubis. Spread your legs a little more so that you can gently swing the weight back and forth between your legs; notice the stretch on the pubis as it swings back. That's sufficient for your first time. It is tempting to continue – but don't - you are going through a steep learning curve – and your penis is too.

Remove the weight and clamp, take off the wrap (if the last bit that's touching the skin stings as you peel it away, try dusting the shaft with a little talc before attaching the wrap next time. Dust the skin, not the wrap; if you dust the wrap it will not adhere to itself as you bind. Minutely inspect your penis, the glans in particular. Gently massage your penis to get the blood flowing properly again. If all is well, rest for ten minutes then repeat the whole process for another twenty minutes. That will be plenty for the first day.

If you are going to include jelqing with your hanging routine, warm up after hanging and jelq for 10 minutes or so – your penis will have been put through enough without further stressing. If you intend to have a more intense jelq/squeezes workout, consider leaving it for half a day before commencing. Many students either concentrate on hanging to the exclusion of all other routines or hang and workout on alternate sessions. However, you may discover you're the exception and manage to go into a full workout routine immediately following a hanging session. But do listen to your penis – don't force it.

Now you are familiar with the basics, you can add half a kilo (1 lb) a week. You can also hang for 30 minutes at a time – never, at any stage, hang for more than 30 minutes without removing the clamp and wrap and encourage the blood flow to return to normal by gently massaging. On this basis you can increase time spent hanging week by week; it is a time consuming routine. The most successful guys that shared their discoveries and secrets with me worked at home, mostly at a desk and uninterrupted. How you spend your day will largely dictate the number of hours you can dedicate to hanging.

How much weight, and what angles?

I concur with correspondent, 'Bigger', when asked this question: 'I'm wary of giving weight recommendations ... can only speak for myself

... we are all individual's and our reactions to differing weights, time spent, postures adopted, vary greatly.'

By way of explaining so that you can appreciate some of the elements that must enter the equation, and thereby help you make your own personal decisions, I'm going to reproduce here the relevant text of an email I sent to another correspondent when I had been hanging weights for a couple of months with a home-made penis clamp and decided to invest in a professional model:

'.......new hanger arrived today. So, this afternoon, warmed up for 6/7 minutes. Stretched out penis and clamped on hanger, as high up penis as I could – leaving glans, covered by foreskin, exposed. Used two pieces of soft toilet tissue as a comfort wrap. Attached 12 lb (5.4 kilo) weight. Sat on edge of bathtub, facing out, and let penis hang while getting used to hanger and weight.

Slight discomfort at first but this feeling went after 2/3 minutes. Noticed that skin over pubic area was tight as a drum, particularly at sides where pubis meets thighs. Impression was that weight had to stretch not just the ligament but skin, too. Five minutes into hanging and getting a little more comfortable. Stood up and tried moving weight in circles and pendulum motions – felt good. After 15 minutes was able to experiment with other positions. Stood as though about to touch toes but with knees bent, so that I was looking directly at genitals. Felt a change in the direction of pull.

After a few minutes of this I sat down again, with feet spread and weight hanging straight down. This became a rest position, between variations, to prevent boredom. Next, from this rest position, placed hands either side of me onto the rim of the bath, to take body weight. With torso upright, raised body so that my bottom was as high as I could get – and pointed feet so that only toes remained on the floor. The weight was now hanging at almost optimum down position. Then tensioned stomach muscles – aimed for a flat tummy – and felt the extra stretch immediately! Put my feet firmly back on the floor and swung weight to and fro, like a pendulum, between knees and buttocks. I did all the foregoing for 30 minutes, removed the hanger and saw virtually no stress marks. 2/3 minutes of warm water wash while massaging. Because I felt that all the stretching had been on the upper (pubic) end of the ligament, I then did 5 minutes of manual stretches and it definitely felt like my penis had not been stretched lengthwise, which, to my mind, does confirm something about the opposing ends of the ligament strands.'

Just a reminder at this point: **do not start this way** – don't forget I had been practising hanging for some months before I reached this point. From the foregoing you will have gained enough to begin your own trial hanging sessions. As indicated earlier, I'm going to take this section further, not by telling you what to do but, by using the question/answer technique, help you benefit from the answers given by 'Bigger', my experienced correspondent, to students who not only posed the questions but also advised (in most instances) what routines they were following:

Q: *How do I tell if I'm overworking? After my workouts I only feel a little soreness in the ligaments when I push against my pubic bone. Apart from that, just a little tenderness in the skin.*

A: *That is almost exactly the way I would describe how you should feel after a workout. You should be fatigued in the shaft from time to time. Overworking would be hanging at a higher weight, having erection failure, head problems (like numbness), or any* <u>pain</u> *in the area after workout.*

Q: *There are times when I'll hook up 10-12 lbs (4.5-5.4 kilos) and feel like I couldn't add another pound – usually from skin pulling or pressure points – but after I've finished I hardly feel worked out enough. Other times I'll hang 20-25 lbs (9-11.3 kilos) and it feels very comfortable and bearable and I get a good stretch. I know I* *moved up (in weights) rather quickly but to get any kind of worked out feeling I need the heavy weight.*

A: Firstly, the feelings about how much you can handle are not unusual. Secondly, what you have to do in hanging is drive towards stressing the areas which gain most from the stresses. The skin is easy to stretch, but can be limiting until it is (stretched). The area you wrap and the position of the hanger will affect how much the skin is stretched. You may have to hang heavier weights for a period to get the ligaments and shaft moving. Then you may discover that you cannot hang this maximum weight for a day or two, or even longer. A lower weight may give good stresses for this period because, with the tougher ligaments taken care of, the remaining are not as tough. So, you need to remember there are many of these situations in micro-areas all through the ligaments and shaft components. In talking with others, it seems that the need to lower weight is a good sign. Sometimes described as an 'electric' feeling, it seems that good stretches occur during these periods. <u>The key is not to push things and over work</u>. When you simply cannot hang your maximum weight, or there is any kind of discomfort, bring the weight down. If you have to move down to less than one half your maximum weight, then stop in order to avoid overstress. <u>Don't fight it!</u>

Using heat will ensure you will be stressing pliable tissues and help avoid overstress. It will also give more results with an equal amount of work. Also be aware that, when you change angles of hang, this will present new stresses that will require thinking about when considering weight used. The only one who knows how much weight to use is the individual hanger. There are times when lower weights for longer periods is more beneficial than heavy weight for shorter periods. The secret is whether or not you can feel the stress.

If you can't, then change because you are probably wasting your time.

Lastly, check that you're not limited in weights used by hanger attachment problems. Pinching or any pain from the hanger is counter-productive and can influence your perception of stresses. As I always say, the best thing you can do in PE is become attuned to what you are feeling. Learn to read these feelings; know exactly where they are and why they are occurring. If there is a hanger problem, fix it before going any further.

Q: *Erection problems. It seems like I never get 100% hard any more. I have been mainly hanging and only jelq occasionally now. When I first started, jelqing only, I would wake out of sleep with rock hard erections. Not so since hanging.*

A: *This is a difficult area to diagnose; another reason why I'm wary of giving weight recommendations. I had softer erections but always in a period of gain. This could last for a couple of weeks. But I also had erection problems from abuse due to bad hangers (bruising) or over stressing. When you stress/stretch your penis, you are also stressing/stretching the nerves. If you have any growth, you must be aware that the nerves involved must also be changing, at least to a certain extent. Using common sense, the nerves will also be a limiting factor. So, if you ever have erection problems due to decreased sensitivity, you must take time off until things return to normal.* <u>No question.</u>

These areas are the toughest things to talk about in PE because they go directly to the risk/reward relationship. Everyone must realise that this is an individual thing.

Warning Signs (a continuation of the forum discussion).

First, continue to remember to be patient. Hanging a roll of duct tape is good. Get the kinks worked out first. Warning signs: there are two classes, three kinds, two are bad and one is good!

First are the stresses that are unrelated to enlargement. These are skin irritation, trauma to nerves, vessel damage, bruises, red spots, etc. These are caused by faulty equipment, improper attachment or overworking. They are bad, but some of this will occur no matter what. Try to limit the amount of blood in the head before attaching the hanger. Be sure the skin is not 'bunched' under the wrap. There should be no pain while hanging. Make sure the hanger has no sharp edges and that no part of it is actually in contact with the skin. Make sure no part of the hanger rides on the top of the shaft, immediately behind the head. If, while hanging, something does not feel right, stop. Take off the hanger and milk to return full circulation.

Second, are stresses which cause the enlargement; stretch marks on the skin, ligament soreness, shaft soreness, general genital fatigue. This means you are working, getting a good stretch, and making progress. DO NOT attempt to increase the workload (time/weight) as long as you feel this. Be sure to rest enough to allow for recovery.

Last, are stresses from overwork? This includes pulled or ruptured ligaments, torn tunica, severe bruising. These occur when you lose patience, increase the work load too quickly, and have an accident while hanging, and so on.

Q: *Is it normal for the head to swell up to almost erection size while the shaft stays flaccid?*

A: *'No. The head should not swell much while hanging, even at 5 lbs (2.25 kilos) or so. The weight alone is usually enough to restrict blood flow – in and out – also the hanger will be tight enough to limit this when you hang.*

Q: *What change of colours are bad; my head went from dark red to a light blue with shades of purple. Is this bad?*

A: *Yes. Any time your head (the glans) becomes dark take off the hanger and restore circulation. Slight skin colouring is okay, but keep an eye on it. You had a situation where the inflow of blood was not restricted, but the outflow was. The wrapping and hanger prevented any blood from leaving the head.*

Q: *How can I be sure that the shaft is taking most of the weight? I felt the sensation throughout the whole organ, including the head.*

A: *Practise. There's definitely a learning curve to hanging. Experiment with different tightness' and hanger placement. You will learn to feel when the pressure is on the head, or the shaft, or both. There should be no discomfort around the head. You may have some discomfort in the shaft and base area from the stretch. It should not be severe. If it is, stop!*

Q: *I hear people talking about 15 minutes but all three time I tried I had to remove it after ten. Why?*

A: *This is not unusual. As your body adjusts, your penis will become 'stronger' – you will be able to increase time and weight as this occurs.*

Angles (the discussion continues)

Q: *I've noticed that hanging weights in different directions limits the amount of weight and causes stresses that are unique to that 'posture'. Currently, I only have the time and energy to hang 5 days per week, and then for only 3 sets of 20 minutes, yet the ligaments in my pubic area and main ligament in the shaft are sore. That* *being the case, what would give me the best/most efficient workout for such a limited schedule? Right now I hang for 2 sets of 20 minutes (16 lbs – 7.25 kilos) straight down, and one set of 20 minutes (10 lbs -4.5 kilos) BTC (between the cheeks). I also have questions about how certain hang directions stress my member. Let's say I was going to hang a certain way, and only that way, for the next 12 months, what would my results probably be? What would happen if I only hung straight down while standing every time? What would happen if I hung over my shoulder every time? What would happen if I hung only BTC every time?*

A: *There are several ways to look at these questions. One is the practical, day-to-day, occurrences. Another is the physical changes. Then there are the straight engineering factors. All have to be considered.*

Think of the pubic area from a strictly engineering point of view. The tunica, which surrounds the blood cavities, is very tough – like hard rubber – and long. It is anchored in the body close to the prostate. There are different amounts of penis, and therefore tunica, held within the body. This is held in by the ligaments attached to the pubic bone – fan shaped – and the tunica on the shaft. Almost like a boom on a crane when erect. The ligaments are like rope bundles; some of the strands are long, and some shorter. The shorter the fibre, the more stress that fibre takes in an erection. The penis is anchored firmly within the body.

Also in this system are blood vessels (plumbing) and nerves (communications). The goal is to pull out as much tunica as is possible – easy, fast gains – by stretching the ligaments, and also to stretch the tunica and associated structures – harder gains. These other structures, corpus cavernosa, blood vessels, nerves, skin, etc.; all are easily stretched. The limiting factors are the tunica and ligaments.

Another goal is to stretch the tough infrastructure without damaging the plumbing or communications. The blood vessels are tough (tear resistant), but easily stretched. The only problem associated with them is the fact that they become narrower as they are stretched, thereby limiting blood flow. The nerves are easily stretched – and also easily broken – but most times regenerate over time. One good reason for taking things slowly is to give the nerves time to regenerate. As long as there are <u>small</u> gaps or tears in the nerves, they have no problem rebuilding. When the gaps become large is the time one experiences a loss of feeling.

The tunica is fairly consistent, tough, and slow to stretch. It takes time and perseverance. The ligaments vary in toughness; you may have several short, but thin, fibres which are easily broken and/or stretched. This will give fast gains. Or you may have short, thick, fibres which are hard to break or stretch immediately (tough gainers). Once these short, thick, fibres are broken, gains may be easy. Then, later, the longer fibres come into play or, as I should say, as the shorter ones are broken or stretched, the longer ones increasingly come into play. As time goes on, more and more fibres are involved at the same time during the stretch. Short ones break or stretch, and the next shortest take more of the load. <u>This is why gains eventually slow down for everyone.</u> This is also one reason why it takes increasingly higher weights to achieve gains. It is also why some people talk about the ligaments becoming tougher. They are somewhat tougher because they become thicker as they heal. But, more than that, each fibre becomes more equal with the other fibres as time goes on; they increasingly resist the stretch in harmony.

At this point, one must become more refined in the attack. Vary the angles even more. For example, after hanging for several months, a good stress is to hang under each leg, over the side edge of the chair while seated in an almost BTC position. This greatly stresses each <u>side</u> of the ligament bundle – dividing and conquering! Then a normal BTC hang will stress the middle of the bundle. The sides are already longer from the side stretch – so the middle then has to take the load. This is just one example.

Limiting Factors

Each micron of gain is dependent upon breaking the next limiting factor. That next limiting factor may be large or small. This is an argument for going up in weight quickly. Break or stretch each limiting factor before the preceding limiting factor has time to heal and become tougher as a result. But it is a balancing act between gaining and being safe. The relative soreness or fatigue in an area is an indication of what has transpired. If you are very sore in an area, you have pushed it far enough. You need to work on another area for a while (a day or two).

Changes in the limiting factors are also a reason you have to go down in weight from time to time. Your current limiting factor may be one or more tough thick ligament fibres, for example. Then, as your maximum weight goes up, one day these fibres fail. When they do you achieve gains, but also incur the next limiting factors. These next limiting factors may be thinner, or fewer, and require somewhat less weight to break or stretch. That is why, from time to time, you just cannot hang the maximum, at a certain angle, that you could previously.

Look at a broad example: you have the tunica hanging straight down then, on top of that, the ligaments are attached, also hanging straight down. Now apply a stress to them. Which structure takes the stress first? It depends on their individual lengths.

For most, if not all, it is the bundle of ligaments – the shorter ones first. So, when hanging straight down or BTC, the tunica may not be *affected at all, taking none of the stress. Only the ligaments. Now, as the angle rises, say, to hanging straight out, the ligaments take less and less stress and the tunica take more and more. Thus, when hanging straight up (over the shoulder), most, if not all, will have all the stress on the tunica and the anchor points within the body, and none on the ligaments. Further, hanging over the legs will stress the sides of the tunica and the anchor points within the body on each side.*

The tunica and each individual fibre of the ligaments all have different load capacities. All are subject to a maximum load factor, above which they will fail. When they fail they either stretch or are broken. In either case the body subsequently repairs them. <u>This repair time varies between fibres and individuals.</u> *The key is to control the damage done to the structures and allow time for repair. In order to do this efficiently, the best way would be one at a time. Obviously, this is not possible but the varying angles of stress will allow the most efficient method of stressing individual fibres and thereby achieving the goals.*

The best approach

So now we know the problems and what needs to be done. What is the best way to go about it? It depends on the individual, and what has transpired before. If you are very sore in the pubic bone area (the ligaments), it is time to work on the tunica and anchor points. This means over the shoulder, and legs, or straight out, 90 degrees from the body. If the tunica (shaft) and area above the testicles is sore, it is time for straight down or BTC.

The foregoing is very generalized. There are sub-categories of stresses that can be applied to give the most efficient types of work.

All of the preceding *italicised* text was taken from 'Thunder's Place', a forum discussion between students and 'Bigger' who was a Co-Administrator of that forum at the time. The question and answer period finished with one final note on discolouration of the penis head with a further explanation of the circumstances that cause discolouration and a comment on the design of hangers. I mention this before setting out the final comments so that you should know the responses are made by someone who had/has a vested interest in the manufacture and supply of an established hanger.

Q: *Something that still concerns me is the fairly rapid discolouration of the head, especially when I finally hung 7.5 lbs (3.4 kilos). It was not more than 10-15 minutes before I felt the need to dismount the hanger. I'm not sure how this will translate as I go to even higher weights, but we'll see. It would seem to require even more tightening which may accelerate discolouration during hanging.*

A: *Actually, the hanger is designed to allow for blood flow, even when very tight. The problem with lack of blood flow to the head comes when the hanger is too loose and slides too far down to the head and cuts off all blood flow to the head.*

Let's say you want to hang 7.5 lbs (3.4 kilos). Also let's say the area impacted by the hanger on the head is 1.5 sq. inches, and the shaft takes none of the force. That would be 5 lbs per sq. inch on the head alone. This is enough force to cut off most of the blood to the head.

Now let's say you tighten enough to where none of the pressure is on the head, only the shaft. The shaft well (on his hanger) covers 9.36 inches. At the same 7.5 lbs., that would require 0.80 lbs. per sq. inch on the shaft. Quite a difference!

The hanger has six lanes designed for blood flow. The veins and arteries within the penis have the ability to direct blood flow where needed. Just because the pressure is high on the internal structures does not mean that blood flow is restricted, as long as these low pressure areas are available.

I do not want to attempt to evaluate the degree of discolouration. You decide when it is too much. But I have hung with as much as 40 lbs. (18.2 kilos) without too much discolouration; what I would describe as dark red, certainly not purple. When it goes to purple you either have too much weight, or the hanger is too close to the head, or it is not tight enough.

Finally, after you first put on the hanger and tighten a little, hold the hanger and pull out the head as far as you can while tightening the rest of the way. This will help capture more internal structures for the hanger to attach to. Hope this helps.

Time and intensity

The silence that meets this frequently asked question is because the amount of time and intensity of your work entirely depends on you. No one can give you that information except yourself. Intensity and time are inversely correlated. As the intensity of the work goes up, the amount of time you can withstand that intensity goes down – and vice versa. Your own particular physiology is correlated with time and intensity. The degree of fatigue on any particular day is a factor.

Here are some questions to ask yourself: How much time do you have to devote to PE? How quickly, in general, do you recover from the work? Are you prone to injury? Do you suffer from skin irritation?

Most on this board (web forum) have started slow, at low intensity, and worked their way up to the maximum time they have allotted for PE. Then they work on increasing the intensity of the work during that allotted time. In general, the greater the time and intensity, the greater the gains, allowing, of course, for appropriate rest time for recovery.

[My thanks to 'Bigger' – http://www.bibhanger.com - for the foregoing experienced advices, and to 'Thunder's Place' – http://www.thundersplace.com - for allowing the reproduction in this publication of their copyright material.]

Hanging angles

You have read a lot about the pros and cons of hanging but not a lot about achieving the different 'postures' required to achieve the differing angles spoken of. It goes without saying that privacy is essential; there's a time and a place for hanging. Wherever it is, you can do whatever you need with a simple wooden chair. From sitting on it to standing behind it and using the back as a rest to hold onto while leaning forward. A little earlier, I wrote about sitting on the edge of the bath. If, like me, you choose to do your workouts, and hanging, in the bathroom, here's one final tip: take a wooden chair in with you.

Here's how to achieve a maximum intensive pull on the main pubic ligament – after you have taken, and practised, the advices previously noted. Straight down hang is achieved simply by standing upright. BTC can be achieved by lying on the edge of a firm bed/divan, looking at the ceiling, with the hang straight down between your legs. Better still, place a chair so that you can put your feet up on it and feel the difference. In the bathroom, sit on the edge of the bath with the chair facing you - at arm's length to start with - and then move the chair closer until you reach the optimum position for best bridging. With the weight attached to the hanger, sit on the edge of the bath (just as I described before) with hands on the rim of the bath at either side of you. Now, one foot at a time, raise your legs by climbing up and onto the chair – use the rungs to do this a bit at a time. The ideal height to reach is the same level as the rim of the bath where you're sitting. It doesn't matter if your legs are bent at the knee – indeed, I don't think you could do it otherwise. Now you have the weight hanging between your legs bit not quite between the cheeks. Here's how: raise your body by pushing down against the rim of the bath with your hands, making your arms straight by locking out the elbows – the higher you thrust your pelvic area into the air the closer to your cheeks the weight will go. Your body, in profile, should now look like a bridge, bridging the gap between the bath and the chair, and the hanger creating maximum tension by placing the angle of hang directly between the cheeks (BTC). If you can hold this position for two or three minutes you're doing well. **<u>You do not start this way</u>**! Wait until you feel ready and capable – and start with a low, low weight. The moment you try this you will appreciate what I'm getting at. All the remaining angles can be achieved by using the chair – use your imagination. But take heed of Bigger's experience.

SECTION VI

MORE HARDWARE DEVICES

TRACTION

Traction devices come in various descriptions; penis lengthener's and penis extenders being just two. Having read this far you will have an appreciation of what happens when you apply a stretch to your penis. Traction devices are designed to not only place that stress on the penis but also maintain it – as a weight does, but without the weight – and you can have the traction set to whatever angle you desire, it is not limited to being just straight down, although a bit impractical to have it any other angle if you wish to be discreet about wearing it in company. They provide an extending tension between the body and the penis head. They are adjustable so, as your penis lengthens, you can adjust the traction to maintain the stretch. This is usually achieved by a pair of adjustable bolts secured to a base ring that surrounds the penis at

Traction
- Penis Extenders -

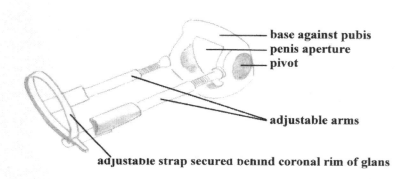

- base against pubis
- penis aperture
- pivot
- adjustable arms

adjustable strap secured behind coronal rim of glans

The above illustration is a simplified artist's impression of a typical arrangement. Although the principle shown is common to all penis extenders, from product to product there are variations in frame design, extension arms, adjustment, and methods of securing the device behind the glans.

the pubis and attached to another ring, or noose, that utilizes the penis head, the corona (rim), as an anchor point to bear against. Attach the unit and adjust the bolts and you have a stretching tension applied. Neat and simple. And if the increasing number of these devices is any indication of their popularity – they clearly work.

However, as with any mechanical device, there can be drawbacks, either in their design or in their application by the student. Only one correspondent volunteered his experience with a traction device, so no claim is made that the following comments are widely held but you may consider his observations. Choice of design, in particular the method of attachment to the penis head, is key to a satisfactory stretch and maintaining that stretch without either slipping off or compromising the glans. Claims are made that such devices can be worn under clothing without interfering with normal everyday activities. This may be true but don't expect to get it right first time; as they say, 'there's a knack'. Just like any other mechanical aid, it would be best applied in the privacy of your own surroundings, without interruption, so that you can 'wear' it for the required length of time and monitor the condition of your penis as you go. As with light weights intended to be hung for long periods, traction devices are also designed to be 'worn' for several hours at a time, six hours a day being suggested as a target time – without interfering with normal and necessary functions, like urinating. The longer you wear it each day the sooner you will see gains – in both length and girth. Remember the effect of avulsions and new cells growing? You can expect girth gains in proportion to length gains.

Our student's trial was limited; he persevered for two months only before giving up. His reported reasons: the penis head attachment kept slipping off when he walked, and wearing it in bed at night was impractical for him. (As a married man he didn't feel comfortable about wearing the device at night – single men would not have that problem). Having an erection whilst wearing the device caused the penis to slip out of its hold – you must wait until the erection has subsided before replacing your penis in traction. If you have a sedentary job, sitting at a desk all day, for instance, a traction device should be fine but if you do manual work you must consider having the device strapped to your leg to prevent it from becoming a nuisance. To be fair to the more commendable outlets that sell traction devices, I should mention that those operating a telephone help-line, or on-line contact, for advice and guidance, provide a better service than those who simply leave their customers to fend for themselves.

In summary I would say that, once you've got the hang of it (pardon the pun, again), you would probably become a keen fan. Certainly traction devices don't require you to set aside time for specific workout routines – they do work, but they are not cheap.

PENIS PUMPS (Vacuum Pumps)

Pumps, or vacuum tubes, are not new. They go back 100 years, but modern designs, incorporating the knowledge of medical practitioners as well as PE experts and coupled with the input of engineers who have to produce the goods, provide a range to cater for all needs. A far cry from the 1950's when Dr Robert Chartham was the first to market his 'Chartham Method' for 'overcoming erectile dysfunction and to promote penis enlargement.' He pioneered the modern vacuum tube – and was mostly vilified for it by the professional establishment. In the 1960's he was involved in penis enlargement trials – unfortunately I have not been able to locate any credible reports on his findings to describe here - and he continued to write on the subject well into the 1970s. Pick up a copy of the December 1973 issue of Penthouse Magazine and you will find an article of his entitled 'Sex Aids'.

Since those days, manufacturers of penis pumps have sprung up all over the world; from the USA to the Far East, from Europe to Australia. The cylinders are commonly made from acrylic tubing, sometimes other forms of plastic. They come in a variety of shapes, sizes, diameter and length. The better quality pumps are cast or vacuum formed; this allows a thicker wall dimension and also enables conical, and other, shapes to be manufactured. Some have graduated length marks moulded in, others are plain or printed. The cylinders are open at one end (the end that you insert your penis in) and reduce to a capped end at the other, terminating into either a plain male small-diameter pipe or threaded to take a screw-in valve snap-connector. Both types take a flexible narrow pipe, usually see-through polythene, which is connected at the other end to the pump. There are basically two kinds of pump, the squeeze bulb and the trigger type. The illustrations show two different makes of cylinder fitted with the two differing kinds of hand pump described. The pump is the hardware that actually produces the vacuum by sucking the air out of the cylinder. It's fitted with a release valve so that, by opening this valve, air is allowed back into the tube thus releasing the penis from the suction. There are other types of pump, from the basic tubular bicycle type to the sophisticated electrically driven and electronically controlled type but, whatever kind of pump you have, they do not have to be powerful as injury is easily caused if using too great a vacuum. More on this in a minute.

How does a Penis Pump Work?

The cylinder is placed over the penis and the air inside the cylinder is pumped out, creating a partial vacuum. As the rest of your body is still at atmospheric pressure, anything within this area of partial vacuum (in this case, your penis) will have those external pressures pushing blood and tissue into the cylinder and expanding to take up the space provided. Unlike a natural erection, however, when blood (only) is pumped into the penis from within and clamped off to keep it hard (erect), placing the penis in a partial vacuum initially encourages blood to flow mainly around the tissues much closer to the surface. Here's where the body's defence mechanisms kick in; for example, when you accidentally knock yourself, around that area of bruising the tissues swell, and if you were to cut yourself at that point, you would see the clear fluid that causes that swelling. That clear fluid is lymphatic, drawn from the nearest and tiniest blood vessels nearest to the damaged tissues. So, the initial swelling produced by reducing the pressure inside the cylinder is, in fact, the result of the body's defence mechanisms going into action.

From the foregoing you will gather that the enlargement can only be temporary. Equalise the pressure around the penis with that in the atmosphere and everything will return to the state it was in before; well, almost. The return to normal takes time, depending on a number of factors which will become apparent as we progress. The growth we are seeking comes from the stretch created each time – each stretch creating microscopic avulsions, just as we have talked about before. As the time taken to return to 'normal' increases with the repetitive use of pumping, so the new growth at cellular level increases. That's the theory.

In practice

The best advice is to use low pressure. Surprised? There are some very good reasons for this. It is only natural in your enthusiasm to pump excessively, encouraged by watching your penis expand and extend its length with each pump. Damage resulting from excessive pumping range from discolouration of the skin (slight bruising) to a full haemorrhage; the higher the vacuum and/or the longer that pressure is maintained the deeper the haemorrhage and the longer it will take to repair. Worse still, you also risk nerve damage, even an embolism (arterial blood clot – requiring immediate surgery). You should <u>never</u> feel pain. A little less severe, but a warning nonetheless, is a swelling, most commonly in the foreskin near the glans, formed by excessive lymphatic fluid at that point. Sometimes referred to as a 'doughnut', it will go down in time but will create a weak spot that easily repeats the swelling in subsequent pumping – rather like a pneumatic tyre with a weak spot that only shows when you pump it up. The answer to that one is give it time to heal, at least 48 hours, and heed the pressure and timing advice next time.

The other end of the cylinder, sitting at the base of the penis, needs careful attention, too. It should provide a good seal with the skin, be comfortable and not restrict surface blood flow in the skin. It should also not allow the skin of the scrotum to be sucked into the tube along with your penis – we'll cover that in a moment by taking size into consideration. Trapped folds of skin can be taken care of by applying a water soluble cream to help the penis slide in easily and also seal around the base. If it is difficult to stop air getting in at the base it is usually because there's a hair, or hairs, in the way. Trim and shave!

Choosing the right equipment

Choosing equipment that is right for you would be more to the point. Cylinder size and type of pump is only the beginning. The design of cylinder should be taken into account; the idea that one size fits all is completely wrong. Thin walled cylinders are difficult to seal at the base of the penis, and are supplied with synthetic rubber seals to overcome this. The seal is mounted around the base of the cylinder and the penis passes through the opening in the seal then into the cylinder. As air is pumped out the seal cushions against the body and grips the shaft of the penis. They are usually supplied with 3 seals of varying size to accommodate penises of differing girth, and a squeeze-bulb to create the partial vacuum within the cylinder. The squeeze-bulb is fitted with a pressure release valve to allow air back in and removal of the cylinder. It's worth bearing in mind that if you attempt to pull the cylinder away from your penis without equalising the pressure (by using the release valve), not only will you find it difficult but you also risk injury; as you increase the space inside the cylinder by sliding your penis away, you will be further increasing the vacuum – possibly to tissue damaging

Penis Pumps & Cylinders

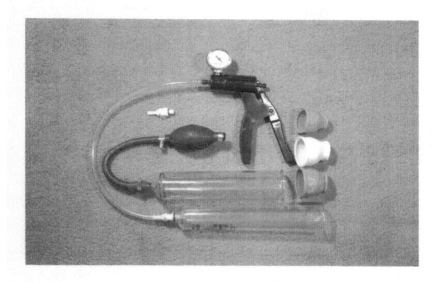

Two of the pumps and cylinders of the types described in the text are illustrated above. The trigger hand pump with vacuum release valve (not in view) and vacuum gauge is shown at the top. At the center of the picture is a squeeze-bulb type with vacuum release valve. Between the two pumps is a threaded snap connector of the type fitted to cylinders allowing the pump and its pipe to be removed from the cylinder without loss of vacuum. The lower cylinder is of the thick-walled, conical shaped type designed for lengthening. The cylinder above it is an example of the thin-walled, straight sided type, requiring synthetic rubber seals to couple the penis with the cylinder to maintain a comfortable seal – usually supplied with seals of varying size as shown, to match variable penis circumference.

levels. So, ALWAYS open the pressure release valve before removing the cylinder. The first illustration shows a typical model of the type just described; it is a basic cylinder, with no snap-release valve but a straight forward push connection for the pipe to the bulb. This means the squeeze-bulb and its pipe have to remain attached to the cylinder at all times. A choice of cylinder lengths is available but little, or no, choice in diameter. There is no vacuum indicator but using a squeeze-bulb is unlikely to produce partial vacuums exceeding -10 Hg. But you will have no idea at what level the actual vacuum is.

The other cylinder illustrated is thick-walled, so no seals are necessary and it bears straight against the pubis without pain, injury, or restriction to blood flow. These models are made to dimensions that fit the purpose, including diameter, whether it is girth or length you are seeking gains in. This particular model is slightly conical in shape, designed specifically for gains in length and to be used alternately with another cylinder of different dimensions and shape to increase girth dimensions. It has a snap-connector valve for the pipe leading to the pump so that the pipe/pump can be removed, leaving the cylinder sealed with its vacuum contained; more convenient if you want to be doing something else while your penis remains in a pumped state, but you will still have to reconnect the pump in order to release the vacuum. The pump itself is trigger operated, with a pressure release valve, and a vacuum gauge.

Vacuum gauges indicate vacuum achieved relative to atmospheric pressure. The symbol Hg represents what used to be a measurement of mercury in inches; 29.5 inches representing the pressure normally found at sea level. This is the approximate equivalent of 14.7 lbs per square inch. Vacuum gauges used with penis pumps are usually graduated in Hg, showing increments of -1 right up to -30 Hg. This allows you to see how much you are reducing the pressure inside the cylinder relative to the atmosphere around you. Theoretically, but impossible in practice with a hand pump, -30 Hg would be close to a total vacuum, like in space!

Coming back to cylinders: there are thin-walled versions that have a flange moulded at the base to facilitate a comfortable seal with the body. There are cylinders shaped to target specific areas, like the glans, or testicle sac. There are cylinders with hooks fitted at the snap-fit valve end, designed to hang weights from while you are pumped up. There are cylinders designed for use in the bath – making use of water pressure instead of atmospheric. The choice is yours but, if you can afford them, the best provide cylinders of the right size, with the best valve systems and sensible pumps. They invite you to submit your erect length and girth measurement and will supply a cylinder to suit. You won't risk having a cylinder, for instance, that has too great a diameter and sucks in more than just your penis.

Measuring up for a cylinder of the right dimensions is simple when you know how. They come in various lengths and I'm sure you don't need me to tell how to choose a length. Be sensible though; an eight inch tube will be fine for most to begin with. Obviously, if you are already eight inches erect, a 10 inch cylinder makes sense. (I apologise for quoting dimensions only in inches for this, but that is the 'norm' in the industry at the time of writing.) You know what your erect girth measurement is (circumference) but you have to translate that into diameter, the dimension used for identifying a tube that will sit comfortably over your erect penis and allow sufficient room for expansion without being too big.

For example: If your girth (circumference) measures 5.75 inches, you divide that figure by 3.1416 (pi) which gives you 1.83 inches in diameter – so you would choose a 2 inch diameter cylinder to allow room for expansion, but not too wide to invite problems of sucking in more than just your penis. If you wanted to work out what the circumference would be from a given diameter, that's just as easy: 3.1416 (pi) times the diameter in inches. Thus a 2 inch diameter equals 6.28 inches in circumference. [For those who might be interested: 'pi' is the sixteenth letter of the Greek alphabet and is used as the ratio of the circumference of a circle to its diameter – approximately 3.14159]

With no apology for repeating some of the foregoing, albeit from a different viewpoint, an extract from an article - or thread, as it is described on PE forums on the Internet – by 'avocet8' at 'Thunder's Place,' that provides an excellent introduction for the newcomer to vacuum pumping. Avocet8 started with a short note to say that he'd made a few changes in his routine since writing this thread, and learned more about jelqing, but here are the basics. (As I've said many times before, PE is continually evolving).

'The equipment you buy is your choice and may be limited by what you can afford. However, when you have an objective such as permanent enlargement, you will want whatever you buy to support your objectives, and that may mean doing some research before you buy anything.

'I did a lot of reading about vacuum erection devices and decided that two elements were especially important to me: a pressure gauge and the size of the cylinder I started with. I purchased a hand pump with a gauge from a company which believes strongly, as I do, that one cylinder size does not fit all and that gains will be more consistent and pumping will be far safer if you start out with a tube designed for the erect dimensions of your own penis. Several pump companies offer a sizing chart and measuring instructions. (Do not cheat guys; your goal is not to impress the pump manufacturer; they don't care.)

'I am pretty paranoid about changing the shape of my penis or damaging it in any way. I like my existing appearance very much, and I also like having good firm erections. While a "show-piece" cock may be a nice locker room device, from my point of view it's got to be one that also goes up and is rigid for sex. Further, I did not want to end up with a "doughnut," a thick, fleshy ring beneath the head – glans - that develops from over-pumping, or even the beginning of one. And, having read posts from a lot of guys who complained of having had painful blisters, abrasions, skin haemorrhages, and odd protrusions of flesh along the shaft of their penises – I wanted none of that, either. I just wanted more of what I had and was looking to augment and get a return of nocturnal erections and firmer sexual ones.

'The pumping schedule I've used is considered very conservative but, as a result of it, I have had no distortions or skin damage. I started this with a 6 inch (153 mm) length and a 5.75 inch (146 mm) girth. By the end of the first 3 months, I had gained a full inch (26 mm) in length and about ¼ inch (6 mm) in girth. Girth [for him] is not as easy to gain as length, and I attribute my own length increase to a careful and very regular program. I seldom exceeded -5 Hg in pressure shown on my gauge in the first months. Most men are comfortable between -3 and -6 Hg of pressure. You will need to find your own comfort level, but do make it comfortable. You can pump 4 days a week and still get gains, but I pump nearly every day.

'Here's my outline; first, the basic procedures: Trim up. A day or two before you use your pump for the first time, it's a good idea to clip pubic hairs at the base of the shaft of your penis, then shave (very carefully) with a safety razor, a narrow ring around your shaft and about half-way down your testicle sac (scrotum) if you are hairy there. Doing this ahead of time will give any tiny nicks time to heal before pumping. The clipping/shaving will provide a clean surface for obtaining a pressure seal with your cylinder rim. In my experience, a few hairs can ruin a good seal. This will not change your pubic appearance much, and a bonus is that it will give the illusion of your penis being longer before you've even pumped once. When you start itching during the day, it's probably time to shave again.

'Prepare your cylinder: have ready, an indelible ink felt pen and a clean, dry wash cloth. Connect the male and female couplers of your cylinder and air tube. Spread a thin layer of lubricant on the bottom rim (or flange) of the cylinder. Apply and spread a small amount of a good, glycerine-based lubricant around the bottom, inside, and two or three inches up into the cylinder.

'Apply a thin layer of the lubricant to the glans of your penis and to the shaft, but not all the way down to your testicles. A slippery testicle sac skin makes it easier to suck one of your testicles into the cylinder under pressure. This is not the end of the world, but it doesn't feel good when it happens. I don't like the sensation at all and it means I have to re-establish a seal before I can continue.

'It's easiest to get an initial seal if you go into the tube erect or semi-erect. You can also pump up if you are flaccid. If flaccid, increase pressure very gradually as you achieve an erection under pressure. Hurrying is not good for your vascular system and penile tissue is very sensitive. When you have a normal erection, you don't achieve that in a mere 20 seconds. Take your time, work up slowly.

'Wipe your hands dry with the wash cloth. Sticky hands make supporting the cylinder or manipulating the handles of a hand pump a slippery problem. Place your penis in the cylinder. With your free hand pull your testicle sac down a bit to accommodate the cylinder rim. Fit the bottom ring snugly against your pubic bone and twist the cylinder a quarter rotation, then back, to create a firm seal. Now you are ready to pump. I think timing is very important in pumping. As you begin to pump, and know that you have an adequate seal, check your watch and begin your timing.

'Pumping feels different from anything else I've experienced. When I did it the first time I was not prepared for the sensations; it all got out of control before I could release the pressure, and I ejaculated into the tube. Semen under pressure has nowhere to go but everywhere within the tube and I was sure for a few seconds that I had blown myself up! Not so, but I learned quickly that I'd have to take a more distant and scientific attitude. I haven't had that problem since.

'The first thing to learn is to understand the difference between pleasure and pain. The line can be very fine. Do not go beyond pleasure to pain, ever, because pain brings tiny skin haemorrhages, major and nasty blood blisters, and flesh distortions. If you bruise or blister, you will have to quit pumping altogether until you heal. [Indeed, all PE activity] There should be a firm sensation of pulling and a pleasant sensation of expansion of your shaft and glans.

'Toward the end of your first session, take your felt pen and mark the outside of the tube with a line indicating the top-most point that the very tip of your glans has reached inside. You will use this as a marker to indicate your gradual progress during further pumping sessions.

'For beginning pumpers, especially, when your session time is up – QUIT – no matter how much you like what's going on in the tube, or how good it might feel to you. You are stretching your skin and the tissue of your penis in ways they have never been stretched before. Do not get carried away with that. Just stop and look forward to the next session. Each time I finish a session, I add some lubricant to my penis and spend a couple of minutes doing massage of the entire shaft and glans, paying attention to all surfaces. Massage has the effect of evening out any blips you may have created by being over-enthusiastic with your pressure or timing and assures complete blood flow, and blood exchange within the penis. Massage will NOT make abrasions or blisters go away if you've overdone pressure, though it may help some in the healing.'

Avocet8 goes on to describe the second part of his regimen, jelqing. He jelqs for 'several' minutes and completes the session just described with a warm down. I have not reproduced that part here because you already know how. He continues:

'Heat relaxes tissue and some believe that heat promotes cell division. This 'break' time usually lasts 5 to 8 minutes for me. I believe that breaks between short sessions are important; newly oxygenated blood enters the penis and with good frequency – this does not happen to any great degree while you are under pressure. If I plan another pumping session, I follow the same lubricating steps as when I began the first session, and then continue.

'Here's the schedule I used, adapted, having talked with sensible pumpers and after reading their advice. These sessions are always at moderate and comfortable pressures. I know a lot of guys are into high pressure and long sessions, but I'd compare my own gains so far with any of theirs.

Week 1: One 10 minute session per day
Week 2: One 15 minute session per day
Week 3: Two 10 minute sessions per day
Week 4: Two 15 minute sessions per day
Week 5: One 20 minute session and one 10 minute session per day
Week 6: Two 20 minute sessions per day
Week 7: Three 20 minute sessions per day

'After a few months I settle on three 10 minute sessions per day and no pumping on weekends. Now I do only 5-8 minute sessions with more squeezes and jelqing between them. I saw no difference in size gain as a result of long sessions.

'A few things to expect: Pumping pressure causes the Cowper's gland to produce more fluid than you would normally experience. "Pre-cum," the clear, slippery fluid you may have during sex foreplay, may ooze into the tube. You may also have some oozing after your sessions are over. Don't be concerned about this.

'It is common for the penis to remain longer and fatter after a session. You have filled it with blood and lymphatic fluids. Your penis will have a "spongy" feeling. In the beginning of your pumping experience this flaccid increase does not last very long at all, but it's fun while it's there. Slowly, over weeks, you will probably find that you are hanging longer and heavier for hours, then all day, then for a couple of days between pump sessions. You are beginning to see permanent gains. Unlike some, I do not believe that pumping gives fully permanent gains. But a minimal maintenance schedule of pumping 3 or 4 times a month will let you keep what you've worked for. That, to me, is permanent enough.

'If you find that your normal, non-pumped, erections become soft or spongy instead of the rigid ones you used to have, you are overdoing pressure or session timing. Cut back. Having good sexual erections should be one of your goals.

'If the frequency of your night-time/waking erections increases after a month or so, or you are more aware of them, you are doing the right thing. They may also be thicker and longer. You may find that you can last longer during sex. It's not that you are de-sensitized; it's just that pumping has trained you to handle more sensation without ejaculating as soon.

'Final Cautions: Do NOT go to pain. Pain cuts progress and causes damage. Limit your session times and be sure to take breaks at least every 20 minutes after you have some experience under your belt. I believe that if you build up slowly, you will build up larger and healthier, from a penile point of view at least.'

When asked about concentrating on length, as opposed to gaining more girth as well, another correspondent, who'd been in the pumping business for 30 years, so I guess he knew his subject, replied as follows:

'The question of lateral expansion versus length expansion is a valid one. Bear in mind that regimens with the objective of permanent change need to include jelqing and the way that a tube affects the tension on tissue does make a difference. Ideally, jelqing should take place during a flaccid or semi-flaccid state and followed immediately by pumping. The jelqing creates a positive longitudinal tissue stretch in the penis's core tissue; the pump pulls that out and holds it. The vacuum level doesn't need to be high; it just needs to provide a continuous lengthwise tension on the member. Time is also a factor – the more time in tension, the better.

'Obviously, the natural shape of an inflated soft object (such as a tissue cell) is round – thus lateral stretch reduces length stretch. At the same time remember that you have far more exposure for lateral expansion than you do for length. For instance, when the tube is filled laterally, the vacuum can only pull on the end, or exposed area, which is equal to the cross section of the tube. When the tube is not filled, the vacuum works on the full circumference of the penis, thus feeling much stronger. For this, and several other reasons, girth is far easier to develop than length. [His experience] To limit lateral stretch, the tube needs to be filled. To make the most of the limited amount of lengthwise stretch available, the tube also needs to be lubricated for the full length of the penis so that side friction, or resistance to stretch, is minimal.'

Now that you have read through this section you will have detected that some views differ from others. There are so many aspects that may suit one man and yet not another. You know enough now to begin your own voyage of discovery, to find what suits you best, but take heed of the notes of caution – a thread that has run throughout.

Finally, to finish this section, and to give you some encouragement, one correspondent told me he gained 1.5 inches (40 mm) in length in 3 months with the following routine: alternating jelqing with pumping, 5/6 minutes each, repeat 3 times. Total time approx ½ hour (plus warm up/warm down time), twice a day, 5 days per week.

SECTION VII

USING THE INTERNET

There are several forums on the Internet where you can join in with discussions on this subject, as well as all other aspects of PE. It not only helps you to note the difference between individuals, and their routines, but it is also good to discover you are not alone; there's quite a 'community' out there. Strange as it may seem, anonymity amongst members of that fraternity has bred a trust, honesty, and closeness among the PE students, the professionals, and writers alike.

There is a natural temptation, especially when you think there must be ways of making gains larger or faster, to look for answers on the World Wide Web. And, indeed, you will find plenty there on penile enlargement but here are some things to bear in mind about cyberspace: there are hundreds of thousands (quite possibly, millions) out there who are keen to learn how to increase the size of their favourite member. There are also many out there who are ready to take money from anyone who is prepared to pay for their advice, and hardware.

Fortunately, there are also many willing to share their experiences free of charge but, bearing in mind we are all different, and what may work for one will not necessarily work for another – especially if the offer of advice is coming from people with only a little practical experience – don't rush into new routines without sensible consideration. It is impossible for you to determine what's right from what isn't, until you have done your research over time. So, by all means join in the forums and chat rooms - but take most of it with a large pinch of salt; don't believe everything you read - and certainly don't believe all the pictures you see.

If you decide to correspond with an individual on a personal basis, be selective, and check them out first with a few simple questions: how long have they been practising PE routines; what was their starting programme? What were their statistics before they began, length, girth, and what changes have they noticed since starting, and how many 'vacations' have they taken from PE since they started? Anonymity encourages people to be much more open and free of inhibitions and modesty, and will readily exchange this kind of information. Most, it would seem, are honest – because of the anonymity – but you will also come across those who, for reasons best known to themselves, are not. And that is where exaggeration can be rife. Even websites promoting PE programmes you pay for display testimonials that are difficult or impossible to verify. If considering such a programme, try to find someone who has bought into it and seek an opinion. You will quickly come to recognise 'models' used by more than one programme or, from the apparently honest and responsible web programmes, pictures of the same incredible few who have achieved unbelievable proportions. And, don't forget, these are picked from a global business. From this observation you will gather that there are not too many 10 inch penises in the world – and who is to say they were not born that way?

A word of caution: make sure your personal computer is well protected against viruses, worms, trojans and all the other nasties; anything including the words 'penis' and 'sex' amongst many other nouns, verbs, adjectives, adverbs and abbreviations alluding to all matters penile, are constantly bombarded by rogues intent on making your PC a mess. Be warned – be protected!

To start you off on your searches, some of the more popular web pages are listed here. This is by no means a complete directory; you will discover others, quite often through links from one to another. To give you an idea of the size of the community you can tap into, at the time of writing this, claimed membership of just the three forums listed totalled in excess of 200,000.

It's very easy to get distracted from your own routine when you read what others are doing. Don't. One of the most prevalent reasons for failing to achieve growth is down to inconsistency of programme. Chopping and changing from one routine to another will get you nowhere. Give it time.

Some useful websites:

Free Forums:
www.Thundersplace.com/; www.pegym.com/; www.mattersofsize.com/

Hanging Weights:
www.Bibhanger.com; www.Redi-Stretcher.com; www.PEweights.com;

Traction:
www.jes-extender.dk; www.x4labs.com; www.fastsize.com; www.proextender.com; www.pmdevice.com/

Pumping:
www.DrJoelKaplan.com; www.bostonpump.com; www.vacutech.com; www.Pumptoys.com

Clive Peters

PE Product Distributors:

www.PenisDepot.com

Reference Sources:

www.refdesk.com

www.wikipedia.com

SECTION VIII

PILLS, POTIONS & PATCHES

There would be nothing easier than popping a pill to make your penis grow; no exercising, no workouts, no pumps, no weights, no time spent when you could be doing something else – like enjoying yourself and indulging in your (next) favourite pastime.

Opportunists with an entrepreneurial flair and a keen sense of human nature know how tempting it undoubtedly is to offer a lazy man's way to a speedy and satisfactory result. Penis Enlargement Pills are advertised all over the Internet; and in more conventional magazines and newspapers too. If they are so widely advertised, surely they must work? Don't be a 'sucker'; the purveyors of these pills know the potential market is so large that there will always be an opportunity to supply, especially as new customers are coming along every day. And who would want to admit that he had a smaller-than-average penis by returning purchased pills with a note claiming that he still had a small penis? Mix a lot of 'hype' with a little knowledge, add an irresistible sales message and you will find men who *want* to believe or are prepared to try *just in case* they do work.

There is also an element of psychology in play; you want a larger penis, and you believe in what you're doing towards that goal. A little (or a lot) of help on the way isn't going to go amiss – you really can believe it's helping; and those are the two operative words: 'belief' and 'helping.' In fact, <u>you</u> will be doing all the effective work, the pills will only add a psychological boost. And to be fair to an increasing number of 'penis enlargement pill' suppliers, many of them provide a PE routine for you to follow (to make sure you do gain something) while you take their pills.

This is not to say that all enlargement pills are a complete waste of time; study their ingredients and you will discover herbal extracts that have a history, going back centuries for some, of increasing male potency. By potency, in this case, I'm talking about the ability to achieve a solid erection and to finish with an impressive volume of ejaculate. But make your penis grow, they do not!

So, if your erections could use some assistance, you might consider taking a supplement. Good blood flow is essential, not only for solid erections but also for effective PE routines. If you are having difficulty in achieving, or maintaining, an erection, overworking (abuse) aside, there could be an underlying medical problem. Don't ignore it and hope it will go away. It's true that PE will give a stronger erection to those men without a problem but if you are suffering from ED (Erectile Dysfunction) go and see your medical practitioner, explain what's happening and ask for a check up, if only to ensure there isn't something more serious going on. By the way, don't lie about possible ED in the hope that the doctor will prescribe Viagra® for you; if you are able to have and maintain an erection, such medication will make no difference. That's right, there's no advantage to be had in that case.

Back to the supplements: you need to study and understand what you are considering taking. Those listed below are just a few of the more common ingredients and you will struggle to find clinical trials to prove, or disprove, claims made for their efficacy. Some may suit you, others may not; only you will know the answer to that – and you would probably have to try them to find out. Constituents of pills, as well as the balance of various ingredients, vary from manufacturer to manufacturer – another hurdle to make a guess at. As we get older some ingredients can be more beneficial, and therefore more effective, than others. In other words, one menu may be useless for one man but satisfactory for another. Then there's the method of ingestion; orally (by mouth) or transdermal. The idea is to get the stuff into your bloodstream as fast as possible and with the minimum degradation. A pill designed to be swallowed with a glass of water has to have sufficient (surplus) material to ensure it survives the stomach acids and route through to the small intestine where it will, hopefully, have enough left of the active ingredients to be absorbed by the body and enter the bloodstream. The other oral type of pill, or tablet, often described as 'soft', is not designed to be swallowed but simply left under the tongue to melt in that position. This is a faster route to the bloodstream – and will be more suitable for some, those with sensitive stomachs in particular. Liquid potions are also available – for those who prefer to drink their supplements. Patches can be a good alternative; transdermal means 'through the skin' and the product comes in the form of a patch which you place somewhere convenient and out of sight. Patches have the advantage of providing a 'drip feed' into the system over time, and by-pass the ingestion procedure; the ingredients get straight into the blood stream. Transdermal patches are growing in popularity with the medical profession for many different kinds of medication. But make sure you know what ingredients the patches have before you apply them.

Another note of caution: without making a thorough study of the subject, you should know that some supplements, herbal or chemical, can interact, sometimes violently, with pharmaceutical medications. If you are on any prescriptive medicine, take professional advice before adding supplements, particularly if you have been diagnosed with any cardio-vascular disease or circulatory problem, angina, diabetes, liver or kidney disease. Even IBS (Irritable Bowel Syndrome) can be aggravated, resulting in loose bowel movements or worse.

Here are a few of the more commonly used herbal and synthetic supplements with just the briefest claims made of their effects on the human body; for more detailed information use the Internet on professional and academic web pages.

Supplements

L-Arginine: A naturally occurring amino acid in the body, it is a key element in the synthesis of Nitric Oxide, without which you would not have erections. As you get older natural production of this amino acid reduces, thus a supplement can help. The composition of seminal fluid contains substantial amounts of L-Arginine.

Horny Goat Weed: Emanating from a centuries old Chinese story about a goat herder who noticed his herd becoming friskier when grazing on a particular herb; apparently works the same on humans – or so the story goes. Increased sensitivity and improved blood flow are claimed for this supplement.

Maca: A South American herb, said to increase libido and improve erections and stamina. Rich in essential minerals, especially selenium, calcium, magnesium and iron; claims for this herb could be due to its high concentration of proteins and nutrients.

Muira Puama: Also called Potency Wood, Muira Puama is another herb from South America, with similar claims as an aphrodisiac as Maca. French trials reported that Muira Puama was effective in improving libido and treating erectile dysfunction.

Yohimbe: Used in alternative medicine to treat impotence and frigidity. Stimulates heart rate and blood pressure. Excessive dosage can cause nausea, vomiting, anxiety, high blood pressure, and tachycardia. (This herb is listed on the United States Food & Administration's "Ingredients of concern.")

Tribulus terrestris: Also known as Puncture Vine, Caltrop, Yellow Vine, Goathead, Bullhead, Cat's Head, Devil's Weed and several other names. Studies measuring effect of Tribulus terrestris in raising testosterone levels widely documented but fairly inconclusive. Loosely translated, Tribulus is Latin for 'a spiky weapon' and Puncture Vine seeds have been reported as being used in Southern Africa as a homicidal weapon!

Ginseng: Sometimes referred to as 'man root'; due to the forked shape of the root resembling the legs of a man. Chinese and Japanese versions. Widely used in Chinese herbal medicine, often used to help men with impotence and sexual problems. Reported to possess hormone-like and cholesterol-lowering effects, promote vasodilation. May worsen side effects of stimulants such as coffee and alcohol. Not recommended for people suffering from depression, high blood pressure, hypertension, anxiety or any acute inflammatory problems.

Saw Palmetto: Described as a tonic herb this affects the endocrine system, while acting as a urinary antiseptic, a diuretic and expectorant. Used to improve sex drive and libido and to treat prostate problems.

This list is by no means comprehensive. Other herbal and chemical preparations that you may read about include Damiana Aphrodisia, Korean Ginseng, Ginkgo Biloba, Avena Sativa, Nettle Leaf, Catuaba, Pumpkin Seed, Liquorice Root, Allium Sativum (Garlic), Tongkat Ali and Ashwagandha. In addition there are proprietary blends that also include colloidal minerals, and vitamin C as well as other vitamins.

Good blood circulation is of prime importance to having, and maintaining, an erection; as I have frequently said before, it is also an essential part of a successful PE routine. From the foregoing descriptions you will recognise that all these substances are designed to dilate the blood vessels and increase blood flow – result: stronger erections.

The best advice is to keep yourself healthy, enjoy a balanced and varied diet, take plenty of exercise, and avoid any substances that narrow blood vessels and reduce blood flow, such as smoking. Alcohol relaxes you, increases the libido, reduces inhibitions but, unfortunately, negates the natural chemical functions within the body that help produce firm and lasting erections. The older you are the more obvious this disadvantage becomes.

Keep fit, eat sensibly, and don't be overweight, don't smoke, and use alcohol in moderation. Sound like a boring life? Not yours; just look at the benefits! One final tip: drink lots of fresh water, every day of your life – it is wonderful stuff.

SECTION IX

.... AND FINALLY

Congratulations! Now that you have read the book, you know what to do. You have measured up, set your goals, and decided on a routine to take you through the first three months. Don't forget to make a note, on the blank pages set aside for your diary entries at the end of this manual, of the date you began and your starting statistics.

Looking back on my research files, I have on record two men who had increased the size of their penis (through PE exercising) and both were known, as visiting patients, to their urologists. One of these men was a doctor of medicine himself. Both reported that their urologist had initially claimed that penis enlargement by natural means was an absolute nonsense: 'a lot of baloney', one said. However, neither urologist could deny what they saw, and handled. One of the neurologists admitted that he was constantly approached by men with small penis's seeking ways of making them 'bigger.' Now he was curious and began wondering if there might even be help this way for sufferer's of Peyronie's Disease (hardened scar tissue in the penis that causes acute bending of the penis when erect – making intercourse painful). Just two members of the medical profession that we know of who have seen the evidence for themselves, but the great majority in the big wide world remain disbelievers. As time goes by more of the medical profession will be making their own observations and, hopefully, one day will be endorsing PE as a healthy exercise – as, indeed, more and more women are when they enjoy the results.

When starting out it is not unusual to wonder how you will find the time for your workouts; if you find it difficult to set aside time you'll have no choice but to get up that little bit earlier in the morning and/or go to bed a little later. If you feel you're not a 'morning person', give an early start a try. Workouts, especially in the beginning, give you quite a 'buzz,' due to the endorphins generated when you begin jelqing, and can set you up for the day. Try it, and see how good you feel starting the day that way. If you do have the opportunity to include two workouts a day in your routine, there's little doubt that you will make quicker gains but I do recommend that you work up to this after the first four weeks. Don't rush into the stronger routines immediately – pace yourself so that there's never any strain – your penis does need time to get accustomed to all this work, and it will respond by taking it all in its stride, but not straight away.

It is also important that you stick to a regular routine – five days a week – be consistent, be constant, be dedicated. Don't expect impossible results in double quick time – you have set out on a path that can certainly take months, possibly years before you reach a goal that pleases you and your partner. The single biggest reason for failure to achieve gains is inconsistency; a haphazard routine, working out on odd days instead of every day, guarantees failure every time.

Join the Web forum pages; don't join in the discussions immediately, just visit and browse. There will be plenty of opportunity for you to join in, but it's always better if you have something to contribute (from personal experience). As I've said before, there's a whole community out there; I prefer to call it a fraternity, because it truly is like a brotherhood. You'll quickly discover those who are respected and those that are a waste of time. PE is evolving all the time; there are other people writing about new approaches, even as you read this. But the basic principles, contained in this book, will remain. You're off to a good start, enjoy the experience, and I hope you achieve whatever (sensible) goals you set yourself.

Hardware - pumps, weights and so on – like penis enlargement pills – can be very tempting, but I strongly recommend that you make the most of 'manual' routines for as long as you can; resist pumping, or hanging weights, at least until your penis has reached the point where you are confident about your workouts and in complete control of stresses applied so that your routine can be seen to be working, and without causing any spots, blemishes, discolouration, rashes or any other signs of over-work or abuse. It is a frequent and understandable problem for 'newbies', as they are described, to be over zealous to begin with. Avoid this, unless prepared for serious damage that can result.

A final cautionary note: don't become a *compulsive, or obsessive,* PE'er. There are men who start out thinking they'd be happy with 8 X 6 (length X girth) and, having taken so long to reach that goal, ask themselves: 'Why stop there?' So they don't stop; PE takes over their lives. They become compulsive about their workouts, and never stop. To such a man I would say: 'Get a life!' A penis is for making love with (apart from peeing through). When it does that satisfactorily, even excitingly, that's when you should stop. You can always make your penis bigger but, once it has reached that size, you cannot make it smaller. There's no going back.

for the UK Edition only

Useful Contacts for Help and Advice on Sexual Matters, other than penis enlargement:

Love Life Matters Free service for female partners of men with ED
Freephone: 0800 092 2421
www.lovelifematters.co.uk

Sexual Health UK Cannot give medical advice but can answer questions on all aspects of ED
Telephone Helpline: 0870 774 3571
www.sexualhealthuk.info

Diabetes UK A leading charity for people with diabetes
10 Parkway, London NW1 7AA
Telephone Careline:
0845 120 2960
www.diabetes.org.uk

Netdoctor Independent health website offering advice from leading doctors and specialists
www.netdoctor.co.ukadvice

Relate Sex therapists and partnership counsellors
National HQ, Herbert Gray College
Little Church Street
Rugby CV21 3AP
Tel: 0845 456 1310

The Impotence Association
PO Box 10296
London SW17 9WH
Telephone Helpline:
020 8767 7791
www.impotence.org.uk

Notes

Start Date:

Start Measurements — Flaccid   :Length   Girth

                               Erect   :Length   Girth

Made in the USA
Lexington, KY
17 December 2010